Ketogenic Diet All-Time Favorites

- Best Keto Recipes Ever For Lose Weight and Boost Your Energy -

[Dr. Dean Chasey]

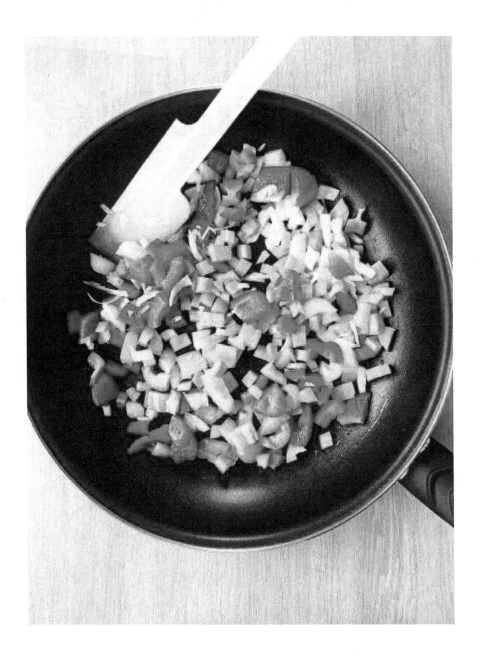

Table Of Content

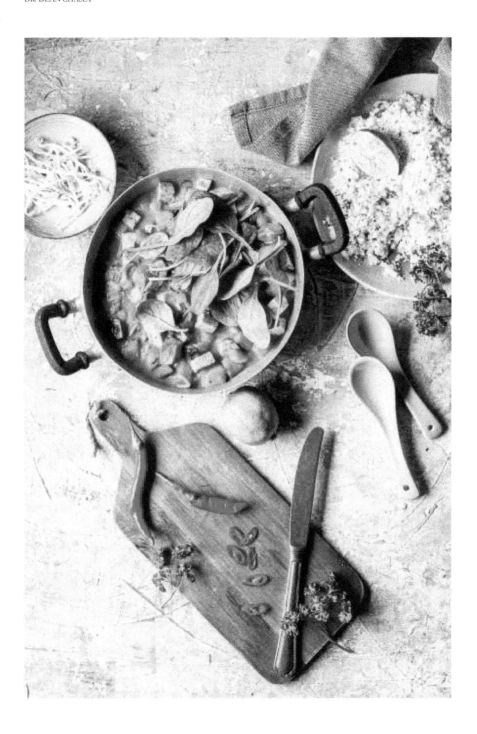

Additionally, the information in the following pages is intended only for informational purposes and should thus be thought of as universal. As befitting its nature, it is presented without assurance regarding its prolonged validity or interim quality. Trademarks that are mentioned are done without written consent and can in no way be considered an endorsement from the trademark holder.

CHAPTER 1: **BREAKFAST**

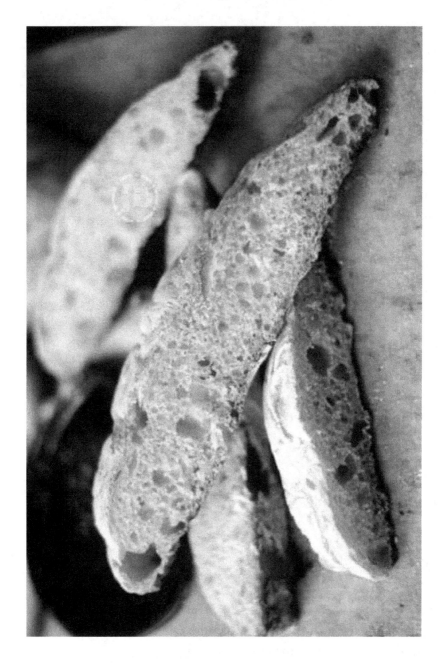

Ciabatta Bread

Prep:

30 mins

Cook:

25 mins

Additional:

1 hr

Total:

1 hr 55 mins

Servings:

24

Yield:

2 loaves

Ingredients

1 ½ cups water

1 teaspoon white sugar

1 tablespoon olive oil

3 ¼ cups bread flour

1 ½ teaspoons bread machine yeast

1 ½ teaspoons salt

Directions

1

Place ingredients into the pan of the bread machine in the order suggested by the manufacturer. Select the Dough cycle, and Start. (See Editor's Note for stand mixer instructions.)

2

Dough will be quite sticky and wet once cycle is completed; resist the temptation to add more flour. Place dough on a generously floured board, cover with a large bowl or greased plastic wrap, and let rest for 15 minutes.

3

Lightly flour baking sheets or line them with parchment paper. Using a serrated knife, divide dough into 2 pieces, and form each into a 3x14-inch oval. Place loaves on prepared sheets and dust lightly with flour. Cover, and let rise in a draft-free place for approximately 45 minutes.

4

Preheat oven to 425 degrees F.

5

Spritz loaves with water. Place loaves in the oven, positioned on the middle rack. Bake until golden brown, 25 to 30 minutes.

Nutrition

Per Serving: 73 calories; protein 2.3g; carbohydrates 13.7g; fat 0.9g; sodium 146.3mg.

Fruit Kefir Smoothie

Prep:

5 mins

Total:

5 mins

Servings:

1

Yield:

1 smoothie

Ingredients

½ cup kefir

½ small banana

1 tablespoon almond butter

½ cup frozen blueberries

2 teaspoons honey

Directions

1

Combine kefir, blueberries, banana, almond butter, and honey in a blender. Process until smooth.

Nutrition

Per Serving: 306 calories; protein 7.2g; carbohydrates 42.3g; fat 14.2g; sodium 127.5mg.

Cacao Nib Nut Pudding

Prep:

5 mins

Additional:

1 hr

Total:

1 hr 5 mins

Servings:

4

Yield:

4 servings

Ingredients

⅓ cup chia seeds

¼ cup cashews

1 tablespoon maple syrup

1 teaspoon unsweetened cocoa powder

1 teaspoon pure vanilla extract

¼ teaspoon sea salt

¼ teaspoon ground cinnamon

5 tablespoons cacao nibs, divided

1 cup unsweetened almond milk

Directions

1

Combine almond milk, chia seeds, cashews, 2 tablespoons cacao nibs, maple syrup, cocoa powder, vanilla extract, sea salt, and cinnamon, in a high-speed blender. Blend until well combined, 30 seconds to 1 minute. Stir in 1 tablespoon cacao nibs and pour into individual bowls.

Cover and refrigerate for 1 hour or overnight. Mixture will thicken as it chills.

2

Sprinkle pudding with remaining cacao nibs before serving.

Nutrition

Per Serving: 202 calories; protein 3.5g; carbohydrates 19.6g; fat 12.5g; sodium 212.1mg.

Raspberry Mini Tarts

Prep:

1 hr 10 mins

Additional:

1 hr

Total:

2 hrs 10 mins

Servings:

8

Yield:

1 - 9 inch tart

Ingredients

1 cup all-purpose flour
½ cup butter
4 cups fresh raspberries
1 (8 ounce) jar raspberry jam
2 tablespoons confectioners' sugar

Directions

1

In a medium bowl, blend together the flour, butter and sugar. Chill mixture for 1 hour.

2

Preheat oven to 375 degrees F.

3

Pat chilled mixture into a 9 inch tart pan.

4

Bake in preheated oven for 10 minutes. Once out of the oven, allow to cool.

5

Arrange raspberries in crust. Heat jar of jam in microwave until it begins to boil. Pour jam over fruit. Cover and refrigerate tart for about 1 hour.

Nutrition

Per Serving: 266 calories; protein 2.3g; carbohydrates 39.1g; fat 12g; cholesterol 30.5mg; sodium 82.1mg.

Herbed Buttered

Prep:

15 mins

Total:

15 mins

Servings:

10

Yield:

10 servings

Ingredients

½ cup unsalted butter at room temperature

2 tablespoons lemon zest

½ teaspoon finely chopped fresh rosemary

½ teaspoon finely chopped fresh thyme

1 teaspoon fresh lemon juice

salt and ground black pepper to taste

½ teaspoon finely chopped fresh sage

Directions

1

Mash butter in a bowl until smooth and creamy. Mix lemon zest, lemon juice, rosemary, thyme, sage, salt, and black pepper into the butter until thoroughly combined.

Nutrition

Per Serving: 82 calories; protein 0.1g; carbohydrates 0.3g; fat 9.2g; cholesterol 24.4mg; sodium 16.8mg.

Mixed Seed Bread

Prep:

20 mins

Cook:

30 mins

Additional:

1 hr 40 mins

Total:

2 hrs 30 mins

Servings:

12

Yield:

1 loaf

Ingredients

1 cup warm water

¼ cup white sugar

2 cups bread flour

1 cup whole wheat flour

2 tablespoons old-fashioned oats, divided

¼ cup coconut oil

1 teaspoon salt

1 (.25 ounce) package active dry yeast

1 tablespoon chia seeds

1 tablespoon flax seeds

1 tablespoon millet

2 tablespoons hulled hemp seeds, divided

1 tablespoon wheat germ

2 tablespoons salted roasted sunflower seeds, divided

Directions

1

Mix warm water and sugar together in a bowl until sugar is dissolved; stir in yeast. Set aside until a creamy foam starts to form, about 5 minutes.

2

Combine bread flour, whole wheat flour, coconut oil, and salt in a food processor; pulse 4 times. Add chia seeds, wheat germ, flax seeds, millet, 1 tablespoon hemp seeds, 1 tablespoon sunflower seeds, and 1 tablespoon oats; pulse until incorporated.

3

Pour yeast mixture over flour mixture in the food processor; process until a dough ball forms, about 1 minute.

4

Turn dough into a well-oiled large bowl and cover with a damp towel; allow to rise in a warm area until doubled in size, about 1 hour.

5

Punch dough down and knead a few times. Form dough into an oblong shape and place in a greased bread pan. Lightly press the remaining hemp seeds, sunflower seeds, and oats onto the loaf. Cover with a damp towel and let rise in a warm area for 30 minutes.

6

Preheat oven to 350 degrees F.

7

Bake in the preheated oven until cooked through and crust is lightly browned, about 30 minutes. Cool bread in the pan for 5 minutes before transferring to a wire rack to cool completely.

Nutrition

Per Serving: 124 calories; protein 3.1g; carbohydrates 14.4g; fat 6.9g; sodium 195.6mg.

Zucchini Quiche

Prep:

10 mins

Cook:

35 mins

Total:

45 mins

Servings:

6

Yield:

6 servings

Ingredients

1 cup biscuit baking mix

⅓ cup vegetable oil

1 teaspoon dried oregano

¼ teaspoon salt

1 teaspoon dried parsley

⅓ cup grated Parmesan cheese

½ teaspoon garlic powder

½ cup grated onion

4 eggs, beaten

1 zucchini, sliced into rounds

1 teaspoon seasoning salt

Directions

1

Preheat oven to 350 degrees F. Grease a 9 x 9 inch casserole dish.

2

In a large bowl combine biscuit mix, oregano, seasoning salt, garlic powder, salt, parsley and Parmesan cheese. Stir in onion, eggs and oil. Mix well and add zucchini. Pour into prepared casserole dish.

3

Bake in preheated oven for 30 to 35 minutes, or until cooked through and golden brown. Let cool for 5 minutes before slicing.

Nutrition

Per Serving: 272 calories; protein 8.4g; carbohydrates 15.4g; fat 20.1g; cholesterol 128.9mg; sodium 635.1mg.

Healthier Cinnamon Spice Donuts

Prep:

15 mins

Cook:

20 mins

Total:

35 mins

Servings:

12

Yield:

12 donuts

Ingredients

cooking spray

Donuts:

½ cup almond milk, at room temperature

1 large egg, at room temperature

1 teaspoon unsalted butter, melted

1 teaspoon vanilla extract

¾ cup granulated sugar substitute (such as Swerve®)

2 tablespoons almond milk, at room temperature

1 cup all-purpose flour

1 teaspoon baking powder

¼ teaspoon salt

¼ teaspoon ground nutmeg

⅛ teaspoon ground allspice

1 teaspoon ground cinnamon

Topping:

½ cup brown sugar substitute (such as Swerve®)

2 tablespoons brown sugar substitute (such as Swerve®)

2 tablespoons unsalted butter, melted

¾ teaspoon ground cinnamon

Directions

1

Preheat the oven to 350 degrees F. Spray 2 donut pans with nonstick cooking spray.

2

Place 1/2 cup plus 2 tablespoons almond milk, egg, butter, and vanilla in a bowl and mix well. Add granulated sugar substitute and mix until well combined.

3

Sift flour, baking powder, cinnamon, salt, nutmeg, and allspice together. Add to the egg mixture and stir to combine. Pour into the donut pans, filling each cavity 3/4 full.

4

Mix 1/2 cup plus 2 tablespoons brown sugar substitute and cinnamon together for the topping. Sprinkle over the donuts. Drizzle melted butter over the tops.

5

Bake in the preheated oven until golden brown, 18 to 21 minutes. Let cool in the pans for 10 minutes, the transfer to a wire rack to cool completely.

Nutrition

Per Serving: 70 calories; protein 1.7g; carbohydrates 30.9g; fat 2.9g; cholesterol 21.4mg; sodium 103.8mg.

Creamy Avocado Pesto

Prep:

15 mins

Cook:

10 mins

Total:

25 mins

Servings:

4

Yield:

4 servings

Ingredients

1 (8 ounce) package penne pasta
1 avocado, peeled and pitted
salt and ground black pepper to taste
½ lemon, juiced
½ cup fresh basil, or more to taste
2 tablespoons grated Romano cheese
2 cloves garlic
¼ cup olive oil
salt and ground black pepper to taste
2 tablespoons grated Romano cheese

Directions

1

Fill a large pot with lightly salted water and bring to a boil. Stir in penne, and return to a boil. Cook pasta uncovered, stirring occasionally, until mostly cooked through, but still firm to the bite, 8 to 10 minutes. Add shrimp to boiling water and cook until shrimp are bright pink on the outside and the meat is no longer transparent in the center, 2 to 3 minutes. Drain penne and shrimp; transfer back to empty pot.

2

Blend avocado, lemon juice, basil, 2 tablespoons Romano cheese, garlic, salt, and black pepper in a food processor until smooth. Add olive oil and pulse until creamy. Remove blade from food processor and stir diced tomatoes into the creamy pesto. Transfer pesto to pot with pasta and shrimp; stir to coat. Serve with about 2 tablespoons Romano cheese, salt, and black pepper.

Nutrition

Per Serving: 480 calories; protein 16.6g; carbohydrates 50.3g; fat 24.5g; cholesterol 50.6mg; sodium 145.2mg.

Blueberry Soufflè

Prep:

15 mins

Additional:

5 hrs

Total:

5 hrs 15 mins

Servings:

12

Yield:

1 torte

Ingredients

½ cup butter, melted

½ cup white sugar

1 (8 ounce) package cream cheese, softened

1 cup confectioners' sugar

2 (4.8 ounce) packages graham crackers, crushed

1 (21 ounce) can blueberry pie filling

1 cup whipped topping (such as Cool Whip®)

Directions

1

Mix graham crackers, butter, and white sugar together in a bowl; press mixture into the bottom of a 9x13-inch baking dish. Chill crust until firm, about 1 hour.

2

Beat cream cheese and confectioners' sugar together in a bowl until light and fluffy, 2 to 3 minutes. Fold in whipped topping.

3

Spread cream cheese mixture evenly onto crust; top with blueberry pie filling. Chill until firm, 4 hours or overnight.

Nutrition

Per Serving: 408 calories; protein 3.3g; carbohydrates 59.5g; fat 17.9g; cholesterol 40.9mg; sodium 256.3mg.

Tofu Scramble

Prep:

10 mins

Cook:

15 mins

Total:

25 mins

Servings:

4

Yield:

4 servings

Ingredients

1 tablespoon olive oil

1 (14.5 ounce) can peeled and diced tomatoes with juice

1 bunch green onions, chopped

1 (12 ounce) package firm silken tofu, drained and mashed

ground turmeric to taste

salt and pepper to taste

Directions

1

Heat olive oil in a medium skillet over medium heat, and saute green onions until tender. Stir in tomatoes with juice and mashed tofu.

Season with salt, pepper, and turmeric. Reduce heat, and simmer until heated through. Sprinkle with Cheddar cheese to serve.

Nutrition

Per Serving: 190 calories; protein 12g; carbohydrates 9.7g; fat 11.5g; cholesterol 18.1mg; sodium 305.8mg.

Croque Madame with Poached Eggs

Prep:

10 mins

Cook:

10 mins

Total:

20 mins

Servings:

2

Yield:

2 sandwiches

Ingredients

6 slices avocado

4 slices Dietz & Watson Maple Honey Ham

2 eggs

1 tablespoon white vinegar

3 slices Dietz & Watson Swiss Cheese

1 English muffin

Directions

1

Cut the top off the English muffin, using the muffin as the base for the Croque Madame.

2

Place three slices of avocado on each muffin base, then place the Dietz & Watson Swiss Cheese on top. Place the Dietz & Watson Maple Honey Ham on top of that.

3

Prepare a pot for the eggs. Fill a shallow saucepan with three inches of water and bring it to a simmer.

4

Crack 1 egg into the saucepan and add distilled white vinegar to the water. Turn down the heat until the bubbles disappear. Use a wooden spoon to make the water swirl, keeping egg at the center of the whirlpool. Cook for 3 minutes and remove with a slotted spoon. The yolk should wiggle, but shouldn't be too loose. Repeat with the second egg.

5

Place eggs over the ham. Poke eggs a little bit to allow the yolk to run down each muffin.

Nutrition

Per Serving: 508 calories; protein 32.5g; carbohydrates 23.9g; fat 27.3g; cholesterol 254mg; sodium 708.8mg.

Pumpkin Donuts

Prep:

15 mins

Cook:

10 mins

Total:

25 mins

Servings:

12

Yield:

1 dozen donuts

Ingredients

Donuts:

2 cups all-purpose flour

¼ cup butter, softened

½ cup packed brown sugar

1 ½ teaspoons baking powder

½ teaspoon salt

¼ teaspoon baking soda

1 cup pumpkin puree

1 ½ teaspoons pumpkin pie spice

2 eggs

¼ cup milk

Glaze:

1 ½ cups confectioners' sugar

¼ cup butter, melted

2 tablespoons water

1 teaspoon vanilla extract

Directions

1

Preheat oven to 325 degrees F. Line a baking sheet with parchment paper.

2

Stir all-purpose flour, brown sugar, baking powder, pumpkin pie spice, salt, and baking soda together in a bowl; add pumpkin puree, eggs, milk, and softened butter. Beat mixture with an electric hand mixer on low speed until combined into a batter; spoon into a donut pan.

3

Bake in preheated oven until donuts spring back when touched, 8 to 10 minutes.

4

Beat confectioners' sugar, melted butter, water, and vanilla extract together in a bowl until smooth. Dip warm donuts into the glaze and let any excess glaze drip back into bowl before placing glazed donut on prepared baking sheet to cool.

Nutrition

Per Serving: 262 calories; protein 3.6g; carbohydrates 42.8g; fat 8.8g; cholesterol 48mg; sodium 303.5mg.

Pecan Cookies

Prep:

20 mins

Cook:

10 mins

Total:

30 mins

Servings:

24

Yield:

2 dozen

Ingredients

1 teaspoon baking powder

9 tablespoons SPLENDA® Granular

¼ teaspoon baking soda

¼ teaspoon salt

½ cup butter or margarine

3 tablespoons brown sugar replacement (e.g. Sugar Twin)

1 egg, lightly beaten

½ teaspoon vanilla extract

1 ¼ cups all-purpose flour

1 cup chopped pecans

Directions

1

Preheat the oven to 375 degrees F. Sift together flour, baking powder, baking soda, and salt.

2

In a mixing bowl, cream together butter and sugar replacements. Beat in egg and vanilla. Mix in flour mixture. Stir in pecans. Drop by rounded teaspoon onto ungreased baking sheet.

3

Bake in preheated oven for about 10 minutes. Cool cookies slightly before removing from pan.

Nutrition

Per Serving: 93 calories; protein 1.4g; carbohydrates 5.8g; fat 7.4g; cholesterol 17.9mg; sodium 83.5mg.

Lemon Muffins

Prep:

10 mins

Cook:

30 mins

Additional:

30 mins

Total:

1 hr 10 mins

Servings:

12

Yield:

12 servings

Ingredients

Muffins:

3 egg, at room temperature

1 ½ cups almond meal

¼ cup coconut sugar

1 lemon, zested

1 teaspoon lemon extract

¾ teaspoon sea salt

½ teaspoon baking soda

½ cup coconut oil, melted

¼ teaspoon baking powder

1 cup fresh blueberries

Glaze:

½ cup coconut butter, melted

½ cup raw honey

lemon, juiced

Directions

1

Preheat oven to 350 degrees F. Line muffin cups with paper liners.

2

Whisk eggs, coconut oil, coconut sugar, lemon zest, and lemon extract together in a bowl. Sift salt, baking soda, and baking powder together in a separate bowl; stir in almond meal using a rubber spatula. Mix egg mixture into almond meal mixture until batter is smooth; fold in blueberries. Scoop batter using an ice cream scooper into prepared muffin cups, filling 3/4-full.

3

Bake in the preheated oven until a toothpick inserted in the center comes out clean, about 35 minutes. Cool.

4

Mix coconut butter, honey, and lemon juice together in a bowl until smooth; drizzle over muffins.

Nutrition

Per Serving: 279 calories; protein 8g; carbohydrates 25.1g; fat 18.4g; cholesterol 46.5mg; sodium 196.2mg.

Zucchini Muffins

Prep:

15 mins

Cook:

25 mins

Additional:

1 hr

Total:

1 hr 40 mins

Servings:

12

Yield:

12 muffins

Ingredients

1 ¾ cups all-purpose flour

1 (8 ounce) container lemon yogurt

¾ cup white sugar

⅓ cup lemon juice

¾ teaspoon baking soda

½ teaspoon salt

1 zucchini, shredded

6 tablespoons butter, melted

1 egg, beaten

1 tablespoon lemon juice

1 tablespoon lemon zest

¼ cup white sugar

2 teaspoons lemon zest

1 teaspoon baking powder

Directions

1

Preheat oven to 400 degrees F. Grease 12 muffin cups, or line with paper muffin liners.

2

Mix flour, 3/4 cup sugar, baking powder, baking soda, and salt in a large bowl; make a well in the center of the flour mixture. Mix zucchini, yogurt, butter, egg, 1 tablespoon lemon juice, and 1 tablespoon lemon zest in a separate bowl; pour yogurt mixture into well. Gently stir yogurt, slowly incorporating the flour mixture until just blended. Batter may be slightly lumpy. Pour batter evenly into prepared muffin cups.

3

Bake in preheated oven until a toothpick inserted into the center of a cupcake comes out clean, about 20 minutes.

4

While muffins are baking, whisk 1/3 cup lemon juice, 1/4 cup sugar, and 2 teaspoons lemon zest together in a saucepan over medium heat until mixture comes to a simmer and sugar is dissolved, about 5 minutes. Cover and keep glaze warm over low heat.

5

Poke each muffin several times with a toothpick; spoon glaze over muffins. Cool in the pans for 10 minutes before removing to cool completely on a wire rack.

Nutrition

Per Serving: 210 calories; protein 3.7g; carbohydrates 35.4g; fat 6.4g; cholesterol 31.1mg; sodium 277.8mg

Yogurt Strawberry Pie

Prep:

10 mins

Additional:

1 day

Total:

1 day

Servings:

8

Yield:

1 - 9 inch pie

Ingredients

1 (16 ounce) package frozen strawberries, defrosted

1 (8 ounce) container frozen whipped topping, thawed

2 (8 ounce) containers strawberry flavored yogurt

1 (.25 ounce) package unflavored gelatin

1 (9 inch) pie shell, baked

Directions

1

Place strawberries and yogurt in blender or food processor. Blend until strawberries are in small chunks.

2

In a large bowl, mix together whipped topping and gelatin. Stir in strawberry mixture. Pour mixture into baked pastry shell and chill overnight.

Nutrition

Per Serving: 246 calories; protein 4.1g; carbohydrates 31.5g; fat 12.3g; cholesterol 1.2mg; sodium 150.6mg.

Chia Pudding with Blackberries

Prep:

5 mins

Additional:

4 hrs

Total:

4 hrs 5 mins

Servings:

4

Yield:

4 servings

Ingredients

⅔ cup whole milk

1 tablespoon honey

½ cup frozen blueberries

3 tablespoons chia seeds

½ teaspoon ground cinnamon

1 pinch salt

2 tablespoons full-fat Greek yogurt

½ teaspoon vanilla extract

Directions

1

Combine milk, blueberries, chia seeds, honey, cinnamon, vanilla extract, and salt in a blender. Blend until mixture has thickened, about 2 minutes. Stir in Greek yogurt.

2

Divide mixture between 4 small serving glasses or jars. Refrigerate for 4 hours or overnight, until thickened and set.

Nutrition

Per Serving: 99 calories; protein 3g; carbohydrates 12.5g; fat 4.5g; cholesterol 5.5mg; sodium 61.1mg.

Salad Sandwiches

Prep:

15 mins

Total:

15 mins

Servings:

4

Yield:

4 sandwiches

Ingredients

2 large green onions, sliced

8 slices potato bread

¼ teaspoon ground black pepper

¼ teaspoon paprika

2 large semi-firm avocados, diced

½ teaspoon kala namak (black salt)

2 tablespoons prepared yellow mustard

⅓ cup egg-free mayonnaise

Directions

1

Whisk mayonnaise, green onion, mustard, black pepper, and paprika together in a mixing bowl; add diced avocado, sprinkle with black salt, and stir.

2

Divide salad between 4 bread slices. Top with remaining bread slices to finish sandwiches.

Nutrition

Per Serving: 466 calories; protein 7.7g; carbohydrates 42.3g; fat 32g; cholesterol 0.5mg; sodium 736.2mg.

Cinnamon Swirl

Prep:

15 mins

Additional:

30 mins

Total:

45 mins

Servings:

4

Yield:

4 servings

Ingredients

10 dates, pitted

⅓ cup almonds

⅓ cup cashews

⅓ cup walnuts

¼ cup raisins

1 pinch ground allspice

1 pinch ground nutmeg

1 pinch ground cinnamon

Directions

1

Line a baking sheet with parchment paper.

2

Place dates in a microwave-safe bowl; heat in microwave for 30 seconds.

3

Blend dates, cashews, walnuts, almonds, raisins, cinnamon, allspice, and nutmeg in a food processor until evenly mixed and easily holds together. Press mixture onto the prepared baking sheet; tightly cover with plastic wrap. Refrigerate mixture until solid, at least 30 minutes. Remove from refrigerator and cut into bars.

Nutrition

Per Serving: 291 calories; protein 6.7g; carbohydrates 31.7g; fat 18g; sodium 4mg.

Cheeseburger Pie

Prep:

15 mins

Cook:

30 mins

Total:

45 mins

Servings:

6

Yield:

6 servings

Ingredients

1 pound lean (at least 80%) ground beef

1 cup milk

1 medium onion, chopped

⅛ teaspoon pepper

1 cup shredded Cheddar cheese

½ cup Bisquick™ Gluten Free mix

½ teaspoon salt

3 eggs

Directions

1

Heat oven to 400 degrees F. Spray 9-inch glass pie plate with cooking spray. In 10-inch skillet, cook beef and onion over medium-high heat, stirring frequently, until beef is thoroughly cooked; drain. Stir in salt and pepper. Spread in pie plate; sprinkle with cheese.

2

In medium bowl, stir Bisquick mix, milk and eggs until blended. Pour into pie plate.

3

Bake 25 to 30 minutes or until knife inserted in center comes out clean.

Nutrition

Per Serving: 319 calories; protein 24.3g; carbohydrates 11.8g; fat 18.9g; cholesterol 165.6mg; sodium 493.6mg.

Keto Vanilla Milkshake

Prep:

5 mins

Total:

5 mins

Servings:

1

Yield:

1 serving

Ingredients

1 scoop vanilla ice cream
⅛ teaspoon vanilla extract
1 cup half-and-half cream

Directions

1

In a blender, combine ice cream, half-and-half and vanilla extract.
Blend until smooth. Pour into glass and serve.

Nutrition

Per Serving: 358 calories; protein 7.9g; carbohydrates 15.4g; fat 30.1g;
cholesterol 98.8mg; sodium 116.1mg.

Asian Country Ribs

Prep:

10 mins

Cook:

9 hrs

Additional:

8 hrs

Total:

17 hrs 10 mins

Servings:

6

Yield:

6 servings

Ingredients

¼ cup lightly packed brown sugar

1 teaspoon Sriracha hot pepper sauce

1 cup soy sauce

¼ cup sesame oil

2 tablespoons olive oil

2 tablespoons lime juice

2 tablespoons minced garlic

2 tablespoons minced fresh ginger

2 tablespoons rice vinegar

12 boneless country-style pork ribs

Directions

1

Stir together the brown sugar, soy sauce, sesame oil, olive oil, rice vinegar, lime juice, garlic, ginger, and Sriracha in the crock of a slow cooker. Add the ribs; cover and refrigerate. Allow ribs to marinate in the refrigerator for 8 hours or overnight.

2

Before cooking, drain marinade and discard. Cook on Low for 9 hours. Drain cooked meat and shred, using 2 forks.

Nutrition

Per Serving: 653 calories; protein 48.4g; carbohydrates 13.9g; fat 44g; cholesterol 176.6mg; sodium 2528.6mg.

Leck Lentil Soup

Servings:

6

Yield:

6 servings

Ingredients

1 onion, chopped

¼ cup olive oil

2 carrots, diced

2 stalks celery, chopped

1 teaspoon dried oregano

1 bay leaf

1 teaspoon dried basil

1 (14.5 ounce) can crushed tomatoes

2 cups dry lentils

2 cloves garlic, minced

8 cups water

2 tablespoons vinegar

salt to taste

½ cup spinach, rinsed and thinly sliced

ground black pepper to taste

Directions

1

In a large soup pot, heat oil over medium heat. Add onions, carrots, and celery; cook and stir until onion is tender. Stir in garlic, bay leaf, oregano, and basil; cook for 2 minutes.

2

Stir in lentils, and add water and tomatoes. Bring to a boil. Reduce heat, and simmer for at least 1 hour. When ready to serve stir in spinach, and cook until it wilts. Stir in vinegar, and season to taste with salt and pepper, and more vinegar if desired.

Nutrition

Per Serving: 349 calories; protein 18.3g; carbohydrates 48.2g; fat 10g; sodium 130.5mg.

Pecan Pie

Prep:

10 mins

Cook:

1 hr

Total:

1 hr 10 mins

Servings:

8

Yield:

1 - 9 inch pie

Ingredients

1 ¾ cups white sugar
2 teaspoons cornstarch
¼ cup dark corn syrup
¼ cup butter
1 tablespoon cold water
3 eggs
¼ teaspoon salt
1 teaspoon vanilla extract
1 (9 inch) unbaked pie shell
1 ¼ cups chopped pecans

Directions

1

Preheat oven to 350 degrees F.

2

In a medium saucepan, combine the sugar, corn syrup, butter, water, and cornstarch. Bring to a full boil, and remove from heat.

3

In a large bowl, beat eggs until frothy. Gradually beat in cooked syrup mixture. Stir in salt, vanilla, and pecans. Pour into pie shell.

4

Bake in preheated oven for 48 minutes, or until filling is set.

Nutrition

Per Serving: 512 calories; protein 5.4g; carbohydrates 65.1g; fat 27.3g; cholesterol 85mg; sodium 272.7mg.

Tea Eggs

Prep:

10 mins

Cook:

2 hrs 45 mins

Total:

2 hrs 55 mins

Servings:

10

Yield:

10 eggs

Ingredients

1 tablespoon black tea leaves

1 ounce Chinese rock sugar

2 (3 inch) cinnamon sticks

4 whole star anise pods

6 whole cloves

1 slice fresh ginger root

½ teaspoon Szechuan peppercorns

1 teaspoon licorice root

1 tablespoon five-spice powder

1 piece dried mandarin orange peel

½ cup dark soy sauce

10 hard-cooked eggs

⅓ cup light-colored soy sauce

Directions

1

Place the tea, cinnamon, star anise, five-spice, cloves, ginger, peppercorns, licorice, orange peel, rock sugar, dark soy sauce, and light soy sauce in a large saucepan. Bring to a boil, then reduce heat to medium-low, and let simmer for 15 minutes. Meanwhile, lightly tap the hard-cooked eggs to crack the shells all over. The soy sauce will penetrate the cracks, and color the egg white.

2

Place the eggs in the simmering liquid, and cook for 30 minutes, then remove from the heat, and let the eggs stand in the liquid for 2 hours off the heat. After 2 hours, drain the eggs, chill, and peel.

Nutrition

Per Serving: 98 calories; protein 6.6g; carbohydrates 5.6g; fat 5.5g; cholesterol 212mg; sodium 1260.7mg.

Keto Oreo Shake

Prep:

10 mins

Total:

10 mins

Servings:

32

Yield:

2 cups

Ingredients

5 chocolate sandwich cookies (such as Oreo®)

1 teaspoon vanilla extract

½ cup butter, softened

3 cups powdered sugar

3 tablespoons milk

½ (8 ounce) package cream cheese, softened

Directions

1

Twist open sandwich cookies and scrape out cream filling; discard. Crush cookies.

2

Beat butter and cream cheese together in a bowl using an electric mixer. Beat in powdered sugar, milk, and vanilla extract. Fold in crushed cookies.

Nutrition

Per Serving: 92 calories; protein 0.4g; carbohydrates 13g; fat 4.4g; cholesterol 11.6mg; sodium 39.1mg.

Matcha Green Tea Pancake

Prep:

20 mins

Cook:

5 mins

Total:

25 mins

Servings:

8

Yield:

8 pancakes

Ingredients

1 teaspoon green tea powder (matcha)

1 teaspoon butter

1 cup boiling water

½ cup milk

1 teaspoon vanilla extract

1 egg

1 cup all-purpose flour

2 tablespoons white sugar

2 tablespoons melted butter

½ teaspoon salt

¼ teaspoon baking soda

Directions

1

Place matcha powder in a bowl and slowly add boiling water while whisking continuously until tea is frothy and matcha is fully incorporated. Refrigerate or set aside to cool.

2

Mix milk, melted butter, and vanilla extract together in a large mixing bowl. Beat egg into the wet ingredients.

3

Mix flour, sugar, salt, and baking soda together in a bowl. Sift into another bowl.

4

Whisk cooled tea mixture into the milk mixture. Add sifted flour mixture to the milk mixture and mix batter thoroughly.

5

Heat a lightly buttered frying pan or griddle over medium heat, but do not let it smoke. Pour 1/4 cup batter into the pan and cook until small bubbles are visible near the center of the pancake, 1 to 3 minutes. Flip and cook on the second side 1 to 3 minutes more.

Nutrition

Per Serving: 116 calories; protein 2.9g; carbohydrates 15.9g; fat 4.4g; cholesterol 30.7mg; sodium 223.5mg.

White Chicken Chili

Prep:

15 mins

Cook:

5 hrs

Total:

5 hrs 15 mins

Servings:

8

Yield:

8 servings

Ingredients

1 (8.75 ounce) jar Dickinson's® Sweet 'n' Hot Pepper & Onion Relish
2 cups shredded mozzarella cheese
2 boneless skinless chicken breasts, cooked and cut into 1/2-inch pieces
16 ounces chicken broth
1 cup sour cream
1 (48 ounce) jar white beans, undrained

Directions

1

Mix all ingredients except cheese and sour cream in slow cooker. Cook on LOW 5 to 7 hours. Add cheese about 20 minutes before serving. Serve with dollop of sour cream.

Nutrition

Per Serving: 403 calories; protein 24.6g; carbohydrates 50.5g; fat 11.6g; cholesterol 43.2mg; sodium 568.4mg.

Mozzarella Chaffee

Servings:

4

Yield:

4 servings

Ingredients

4 skinless, boneless chicken breasts

1 cup dry white wine

¼ cup butter

salt and pepper to taste

4 slices mozzarella cheese

1 egg, beaten

1 cup seasoned dry bread crumbs

¼ cup butter

2 teaspoons minced garlic

2 cups all-purpose flour for coating

Directions

1

Preheat oven to 350 degrees F.

2

Place chicken breasts between 2 sheets of wax paper. Pound each to 1/4 inch thickness. Spread butter/margarine over the inside, then add salt and pepper to taste.

3

Place slice of cheese on breast, roll and close with toothpicks. Repeat with each breast. Dip rolled breasts in flour, then egg, then breadcrumbs. Place coated breasts in a lightly greased 9x13 inch baking dish.

4

To Make Sauce: In a saucepan, melt 1/4 cup butter and add garlic. Add wine and simmer all together. Pour sauce over chicken and bake in the preheated oven for 30 to 45 minutes.

Nutrition

Per Serving: 810 calories; protein 46g; carbohydrates 70.1g; fat 32.2g; cholesterol 193.9mg; sodium 633.2mg.

Coated Shrimp

Prep:

15 mins

Cook:

15 mins

Total:

30 mins

Servings:

4

Yield:

4 servings

Ingredients

1 cup all-purpose flour

1 pound uncooked medium shrimp, peeled and deveined

⅔ cup beer

½ teaspoon salt

2 cups sweetened flaked coconut

1 cup vegetable oil for frying

1 large egg

Directions

1

Beat flour, beer, egg, and salt in a bowl with an electric mixer on low until batter is smooth. Spread coconut flakes in a shallow dish.

2

Dip shrimp into beer batter, shaking off excess, then press into coconut. Place shrimp onto a plate while breading the rest; do not stack.

3

Heat vegetable oil in a skillet over medium-high heat until hot but not smoking, 3 to 4 minutes. Fry about a third of the shrimp in the hot oil until golden brown, 2 to 3 minutes. Allow shrimp to drain on a wire rack set over paper towels. Repeat with remaining shrimp.

Nutrition

Per Serving: 581 calories; protein 25.1g; carbohydrates 54.8g; fat 28.3g; cholesterol 203.1mg; sodium 720.4mg.

Caprese Omelet

Prep:

25 mins

Total:

25 mins

Servings:

2

Yield:

2 servings

Ingredients

2 plum tomatoes, thickly sliced

1 tablespoon balsamic vinegar

1 avocado, cubed

½ cup green olives

½ cup canned artichoke hearts, drained and chopped

2 tablespoons torn fresh basil leaves

salt and ground black pepper to taste

½ English cucumber, peeled and sliced

3 (4 ounce) balls buffalo mozzarella, thickly sliced

2 tablespoons olive oil

Directions

1

Divide tomatoes, mozzarella, avocado, cucumber, green olives, artichoke hearts, and basil between two serving plates, layering them in that order. Season with salt and pepper.

2

Drizzle olive oil and balsamic vinegar over layers.

Nutrition

Per Serving: 631 calories; protein 44.1g; carbohydrates 13.3g; fat 45.2g; cholesterol 108.9mg; sodium 2150.4mg.

Asparagus Quiche

Prep:

25 mins

Cook:

35 mins

Total:

1 hr

Servings:

12

Yield:

2 - 8 inch quiche

Ingredients

1 pound fresh asparagus, trimmed and cut into 1/2 inch pieces
2 cups shredded Swiss cheese
10 slices bacon
1 egg white, lightly beaten
4 large eggs eggs
1 ½ cups half-and-half cream
¼ teaspoon ground nutmeg
salt and pepper to taste
2 (8 inch) unbaked pie shells

Directions

1

Preheat oven to 400 degrees F. Place asparagus in a steamer over 1 inch of boiling water, and cover. Cook until tender but still firm, about 2 to 6 minutes. Drain and cool.

2

Place bacon in a large, deep skillet. Cook over medium high heat until evenly brown. Drain, crumble and set aside.

3

Brush pie shells with beaten egg white. Sprinkle crumbled bacon and chopped asparagus into pie shells.

4

In a bowl, beat together eggs, cream, nutmeg, salt and pepper. Sprinkle Swiss cheese over bacon and asparagus. Pour egg mixture on top of cheese.

5

Bake uncovered in preheated oven until firm, about 35 to 40 minutes. Let cool to room temperature before serving.

Nutrition

Per Serving: 334 calories; protein 12.4g; carbohydrates 12.4g; fat 26.3g; cholesterol 105.6mg; sodium 383.1mg.

Mushroom Frittata

Prep:

10 mins

Cook:

23 mins

Total:

33 mins

Servings:

4

Yield:

4 servings

Ingredients

1 tablespoon vegetable oil

1 ½ cups mushrooms, sliced

½ cup diced yellow onion

4 garlic cloves, sliced

1 pinch red pepper flakes

6 slices Farmland® Bacon, large dice

2 cups fresh spinach

6 eggs

1 cup shredded Gouda cheese

2 tablespoons milk

Directions

1

Preheat oven to 350 degrees F.

2

In medium nonstick pan, heat vegetable oil over medium heat.

3

Add bacon and cook until crispy. Transfer bacon to paper towel-lined plate and reserve. Keep bacon fat in pan.

4

To pan with bacon fat, add mushrooms and cook until well browned. Remove and reserve.

5

Add onions and cook until softened; add garlic and cook for additional 2 minutes.

6

Add red pepper flakes and spinach. Cook until spinach just starts to wilt.

7

Return bacon and mushrooms to spinach mixture and add eggs whisked with 2 tablespoons milk, stirring to combine. Pour mixture into ovenproof serving dishes.

8

Top with smoked Gouda and place in oven. Bake for 8 to 10 minutes, or until eggs are just set.

Nutrition

Per Serving: 378 calories; protein 23.7g; carbohydrates 6.3g; fat 28.5g; cholesterol 328.8mg; sodium 713.9mg.

Spinach Dip

Prep:

30 mins

Cook:

20 mins

Total:

50 mins

Servings:

20

Yield:

1 bread bowl dip

Ingredients

2 (8 ounce) loaves round pumpernickel loaves

1 cup low-fat cottage cheese, creamed

¾ cup fat-free mayonnaise

½ cup nonfat sour cream

1 tablespoon grated onion

1 teaspoon fresh lemon juice

¼ teaspoon garlic powder

1 cup freshly grated Parmesan cheese

1 (10 ounce) package frozen spinach - thawed, drained and chopped

1 (2 ounce) bottle diced pimento peppers, drained

1 (.4 ounce) packet dry vegetable soup mix

3 tablespoons grated Parmesan cheese

1 (8 ounce) can water chestnuts, drained and chopped

Directions

1

Preheat oven to 350 degrees F.

2

Remove the top and interior of one pumpernickel loaf. Cut the insides, top and second loaf into pieces for dipping.

3

Place the cut loaf on a medium baking sheet and bake in the preheated oven 10 to 15 minutes, or until dry and firm.

4

In a large bowl, mix the cottage cheese, 1 cup Parmesan cheese, mayonnaise, sour cream, onion, lemon juice, garlic powder, spinach, water chestnuts, pimento peppers and dry vegetable soup mix. Spoon the mixture into the hollowed out loaf. Top with 3 tablespoons Parmesan cheese.

5

Bake in the preheated oven 20 minutes, or until bubbly and lightly brown. Heat the cut up bread pieces until lightly toasted.

Nutrition

Per Serving: 109 calories; protein 6g; carbohydrates 16.6g; fat 2.2g; cholesterol 6.1mg; sodium 331.3mg.

Mocha Smoothie

Prep:

10 mins

Total:

10 mins

Servings:

1

Yield:

1 smoothie

Ingredients

1 cup crushed ice

¼ cup brewed coffee

3 tablespoons turbinado sugar (such as Sugar in the Raw®)

¾ cup coconut milk

1 tablespoon vanilla extract

1 tablespoon hot chocolate mix (such as Starbucks®)

Directions

1

Blend ice, coconut milk, coffee, sugar, hot chocolate mix, and vanilla extract together in a blender until smooth.

Nutrition

Per Serving: 542 calories; protein 4g; carbohydrates 49g; fat 36.5g; sodium 86.5mg.

Almond Smoothie

Prep:

5 mins

Total:

5 mins

Servings:

2

Yield:

2 servings

Ingredients

1 (8 ounce) container cherry yogurt

¼ cup half-and-half cream

1 teaspoon almond extract

½ banana, peeled and sliced

1 (11 ounce) can mandarin oranges, drained

Directions

1

In a blender, mix yogurt, oranges, banana, half-and-half and almond extract. Blend until smooth.

Nutrition

Per Serving: 239 calories; protein 6.7g; carbohydrates 43.8g; fat 4.7g; cholesterol 16.2mg; sodium 95.5mg.

Matcha Smoothie

Prep:

10 mins

Total:

10 mins

Servings:

1

Yield:

1 serving

Ingredients

1 cup ice cubes, or as desired
1 ripe banana
½ teaspoon matcha green tea powder
1 cup orange juice

Directions

1

Blend ice cubes, orange juice, banana, and matcha powder together in a blender until smooth.

Nutrition

Per Serving: 218 calories; protein 3.2g; carbohydrates 53g; fat 0.9g; sodium 11.4mg.

CHAPTER 2: **SOUPS & SALADS**

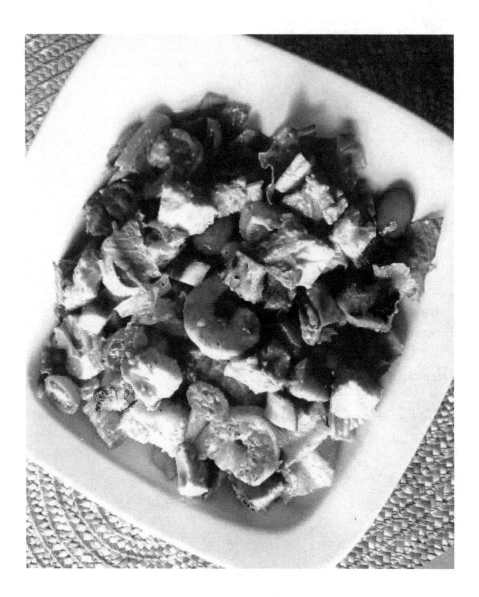

Shrimp Salad with Cauliflower

Prep:

5 mins

Cook:

20 mins

Additional:

15 mins

Total:

40 mins

Servings:

10

Yield:

10 servings

Ingredients

1 head cauliflower, thinly sliced

1 tablespoon minced pimento

1 pound shrimp - cooked, peeled, deveined and chilled

3 eggs

1 cup mayonnaise

¾ cup creamy Italian-style salad dressing

¾ cup sliced black olives

1 cup chopped green onions

Directions

1

Place eggs in a small saucepan, and add water to cover. Cover the pan, and bring to a boil over high heat. Remove from heat and let stand covered for 12 minutes. Cool, peel, and chop the hard boiled eggs.

2

Mix mayonnaise and salad dressing together in a small bowl.

3

To a large bowl, add cauliflower, shrimp, green onions, chopped eggs, olives, and pimientos. Toss to combine. Stir in dressing mixture, and toss to coat. Refrigerate. Serve chilled.

Nutrition

Per Serving: 331 calories; protein 14.9g; carbohydrates 6.6g; fat 27.8g; cholesterol 156mg; sodium 542mg.

Squash Salad

Prep:

25 mins

Cook:

5 mins

Total:

30 mins

Servings:

4

Yield:

4 servings

Ingredients

2 yellow squash, shaved into thin strips
¼ cup crumbled feta cheese
1 teaspoon salt
1 tablespoon olive oil
2 teaspoons fresh lemon juice
½ teaspoon grated lemon zest
1 zucchini, shaved into thin strips
½ teaspoon freshly ground black pepper
3 slices prosciutto, chopped
2 tablespoons chopped fresh mint

Directions

1

Toss yellow squash and zucchini with salt in a large bowl.

2

Whisk mint, olive oil, lemon juice, lemon zest, and black pepper in a small bowl; pour over squash mixture. Toss to coat.

3

Heat a small nonstick skillet over medium heat; cook and stir prosciutto in the hot skillet until crisp, about 2 minutes.

4

Divide squash salad over 4 plates. Evenly sprinkle prosciutto and feta cheese over salads.

Nutrition

Per Serving: 123 calories; protein 5g; carbohydrates 6.5g; fat 9.1g; cholesterol 17.8mg; sodium 901.8mg.

Beet Tofu Salad

Prep:

20 mins

Cook:

45 mins

Additional:

15 mins

Total:

1 hr 20 mins

Servings:

4

Yield:

4 servings

Ingredients

6 beets
1 tablespoon vegetable oil
1 teaspoon prepared horseradish
½ (7.5 ounce) package smoked tofu, diced
½ apple, diced
1 (8 ounce) container plain yogurt
salt and ground black pepper to taste
1 teaspoon maple syrup

Directions

1

Place beets into a large pot, cover with cold, lightly salted water, and
bring to a boil. Reduce heat, cover, and simmer until beets are soft and

can easily be pierced with a fork, about 40 minutes. Drain and rinse under cold water. Peel and cut into cubes.

2

Heat oil in a skillet over medium heat. Cook and stir smoked tofu until hot, 2 to 3 minutes. Combine tofu, beets, and apple in a bowl.

3

Mix yogurt, horseradish, and maple syrup in a small bowl and season with salt and pepper. Pour over salad and mix well. Let stand until flavors combine, about 17 minutes.

Nutrition

Per Serving: 173 calories; protein 10.3g; carbohydrates 20.9g; fat 5.5g; cholesterol 3.4mg; sodium 180.2mg.

Spinach, Pear and Feta Salad

Prep:

30 mins

Total:

30 mins

Servings:

4

Yield:

4 servings

Ingredients

2 pears, cored and thinly sliced

½ cup toasted pine nuts

1 cup diet lemon-lime soda

1 shallot, finely chopped

½ cup crumbled feta cheese

4 cups baby spinach leaves

½ cup raspberry vinaigrette salad dressing

Directions

1

Place the pears in a bowl with the lemon-lime soda. Set aside; this will keep them from turning brown.

2

Place the baby spinach in a serving bowl, and add the shallot, feta cheese and pine nuts. Drain the pears, and discard the soda. Add pears to the salad, and toss to blend. Serve with raspberry vinaigrette dressing.

Nutrition

Per Serving: 299 calories; protein 10.1g; carbohydrates 33.8g; fat 15.6g; cholesterol 28mg; sodium 820mg.

Coconut Cream Soup With Cucumber

Prep:

15 mins

Additional:

2 hrs

Total:

2 hrs 15 mins

Servings:

4

Yield:

4 servings

Ingredients

2 ½ cups coconut water

½ teaspoon minced fresh ginger root

1 ½ cups chopped cucumber

1 tablespoon chopped fresh mint

1 teaspoon chopped green chile pepper

1 teaspoon lemon juice

1 cup fresh young coconut flesh

salt to taste

Garnish:

4 cucumber slices, or to taste

2 tablespoons grated fresh coconut, or to taste

4 fresh mint leaves

Directions

1

Combine coconut water, cucumber, coconut flesh, mint, chile pepper, lemon juice, ginger, and salt in a blender; blend until smooth. Refrigerate until chilled through, about 2 hours.

2

Garnish with cucumber slices, grated coconut, and mint leaves before serving.

Nutrition

Per Serving: 120 calories; protein 2.3g; carbohydrates 11.8g; fat 7.9g; sodium 202.3mg.

Mixed Mushroom Soup

Prep:

20 mins

Cook:

36 mins

Total:

56 mins

Servings:

8

Yield:

8 servings

Ingredients

½ cup unsalted butter, divided

3 tablespoons olive oil

1 ½ teaspoons dried tarragon

8 ounces portobello mushrooms, stemmed and sliced

8 ounces baby bella mushrooms, sliced

8 ounces oyster mushrooms, sliced

3 (16 ounce) cans chicken broth

1 large baking potato, peeled and diced into small cubes

2 tablespoons fresh thyme

1 ½ teaspoons dried oregano

salt and ground black pepper to taste

¼ cup diced white onion

Directions

1

Heat 1/4 cup butter and oil in a large pot over medium heat until butter melts, 1 to 2 minutes. Add onion; cook and stir until soft, about 5 minutes. Add remaining 1/4 cup butter, portobello mushrooms, baby bella mushrooms, and oyster mushrooms, and tarragon; cook and stir until tender, 6 to 8 minutes.

2

Stir chicken broth, potato, thyme, and oregano into the pot. Bring to a boil; let soup simmer until potato is tender, 15 to 20 minutes.

3

Remove soup from heat and puree with an immersion blender until smooth.

4

Return soup to heat and simmer until heated through, about 5 minutes. Stir in heavy cream. Season with salt and pepper.

Nutrition

Per Serving: 260 calories; protein 4.3g; carbohydrates 10.9g; fat 22.8g; cholesterol 55.2mg; sodium 863.2mg.

Thyme Asparagus Soup

Prep:

20 mins

Cook:

20 mins

Total:

40 mins

Servings:

4

Yield:

4 servings

Ingredients

1 tablespoon olive oil

2 dashes dried thyme

2 small onions, chopped

3 cups vegetable broth

½ cup chopped mushrooms

1 teaspoon minced garlic

1 bunch asparagus, trimmed and coarsely chopped

1 dash ground black pepper

½ cup heavy cream

Directions

1

Heat olive oil in a saucepan over medium heat. Add onions, mushrooms, and garlic; cook and stir until onions soften, about 5 minutes. Add asparagus, wine, thyme, and black pepper; cook and stir until asparagus is tender, about 5 minutes. Pour in 2 cups broth. Simmer soup until flavors combine, 5 to 10 minutes.

2

Puree soup with an immersion blender until smooth. Stir in cream. Thin soup with remaining stock to desired consistency and simmer until heated through, 5 to 10 minutes.

Nutrition

Per Serving: 215 calories; protein 4.7g; carbohydrates 13.9g; fat 15g; cholesterol 40.8mg; sodium 362.2mg.

Chilled Tomato & Avocado Soup

Prep:

20 mins

Additional:

2 hrs

Total:

2 hrs 20 mins

Servings:

6

Yield:

6 servings

Ingredients

1 ripe tomato, peeled and quartered

cayenne pepper to taste

2 large avocados - peeled, pitted, and sliced

1 small onion, quartered

¼ cup fresh lemon juice

1 quart tomato juice

1 ¼ cups plain nonfat yogurt

salt to taste

¼ cup chopped fresh chives

1 green bell pepper, chopped

Directions

1

Place tomato, avocados, onion, green bell pepper, and lemon juice into the bowl of a food processor, and process until smooth. Pour in 1 cup tomato juice, and process to blend.

2

Transfer mixture to a large bowl, and mix in remaining tomato juice and 1 cup yogurt. Season to taste with salt. Chill for 2 hours.

3

Serve in bowls garnished with dollops of yogurt, chives, and a sprinkling of cayenne pepper.

Nutrition

Per Serving: 215 calories; protein 5.8g; carbohydrates 22.7g; fat 14.1g; cholesterol 1mg; sodium 663.8mg.

Kale Soup

Servings:

12

Yield:

12 servings

Ingredients

1 medium onion, chopped

1 pound Portuguese chourico, broken into large chunks

3 cloves garlic, minced

4 tablespoons olive oil

2 (15 ounce) cans kidney beans, drained

1 (15 ounce) can garbanzo beans, drained

2 pork chops

salt and pepper

3 tablespoons Pimenta Moida (Portuguese hot chopped peppers)

1 bunch kale - washed, dried, and shredded

5 Yukon Gold potatoes, cubed

½ head savoy cabbage, shredded

Directions

1

In a large soup pot, cook onion and garlic in olive oil over medium heat until soft. Mix in choirico, beans, and potatoes, and then add pork chops to the pot. Season with salt and pepper, and add enough water to the pan to cover all of the ingredients. Bring to a boil, then reduce heat, and simmer until potatoes are tender.

2

Once potatoes are tender, taste soup, add Pimenta Moida and more salt and pepper. Stir in kale and cabbage, and increase heat to gently boil. Kale only needs about 5 minutes. You may add some water if the soup got too thick, I like this soup on the brothy side.

Nutrition

Per Serving: 348 calories; protein 17.3g; carbohydrates 33g; fat 17.1g; cholesterol 36.4mg; sodium 617.7mg.

White Bean Salad

Prep:

10 mins

Total:

10 mins

Servings:

4

Yield:

4 servings

Ingredients

Dressing:

2 tablespoons cider vinegar

½ teaspoon sugar

¼ cup extra-virgin olive oil

1 tablespoon Dijon mustard

Salt and ground black pepper to taste

Salad:

1 (16 ounce) can whole beets, well drained, halved

½ cup reduced-fat crumbled blue cheese

½ cup coarsely chopped walnuts, toasted

Baby arugula leaves

1 (15 ounce) can white kidney beans (cannellini), drained

Directions

1

Prepare dressing: In small bowl combine cider vinegar, Dijon mustard and sugar. Gradually add olive oil until well blended. Season with salt and pepper.

2

Prepare Salad: In large bowl combine beets and white kidney beans; toss with dressing.

3

To serve, place arugula leaves on platter or in serving bowl; top with beet mixture. Sprinkle with crumbled blue cheese and walnuts.

Nutrition

Per Serving: 394 calories; protein 11.6g; carbohydrates 26.3g; fat 27.4g; cholesterol 9mg; sodium 800.9mg.

Chicken Vegetable Soup

Prep:

15 mins

Cook:

1 hr 15 mins

Total:

1 hr 30 mins

Servings:

4

Yield:

4 servings

Ingredients

1 cup chicken broth

1 cup chopped carrot

4 potatoes, cubed

1 (15 ounce) can green beans

¼ cup chopped green bell pepper

1 cup tomato juice

1 cup shredded cabbage

3 cloves garlic, minced

½ onion, chopped

½ teaspoon dried oregano

1 tablespoon dried basil

1 cup cooked and cubed chicken

½ teaspoon Italian-style seasoning

salt and pepper to taste

Directions

1

In a large pot over high heat, combine the chicken broth, cabbage, carrots, potatoes, onion, green beans, green bell pepper, tomato juice, garlic, oregano, basil and Italian-style seasoning.

2

Bring to a boil, reduce heat to low and simmer for 1 hour, or until all vegetables are tender.

3

Add the chicken and simmer for 15 more minutes. Season with salt and pepper to taste.

Nutrition

Per Serving: 317 calories; protein 18.6g; carbohydrates 51.1g; fat 4.9g; cholesterol 29mg; sodium 719.7mg.

Escarole Soup

Prep:

10 mins

Cook:

20 mins

Total:

30 mins

Servings:

14

Yield:

3 1/2 quarts

Ingredients

1 tablespoon olive oil

2 (15 ounce) cans cannellini beans, rinsed and drained

2 (32 ounce) cartons chicken broth

1 head escarole, chopped

1 (15 ounce) can tomato sauce

2 pounds bulk Italian sausage

Directions

1

Heat the olive oil in a stockpot over medium heat. Cook the sausage in the oil until evenly browned, 6 to 10 minutes. Add the chicken broth, beans, escarole, and tomato sauce; simmer another 15 to 20 minutes.

Nutrition

Per Serving: 303 calories; protein 16.4g; carbohydrates 15g; fat 19.4g; cholesterol 40.2mg; sodium 1688.1mg.

CHAPTER 3: LUNCH

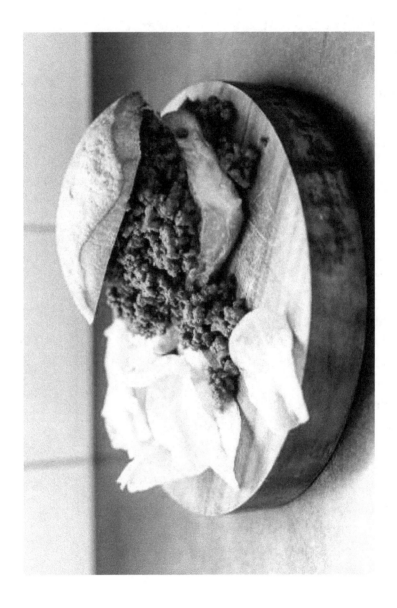

Sloppy Joes

Prep:

20 mins

Cook:

25 mins

Total:

45 mins

Servings:

5

Yield:

5 sandwiches

Ingredients

1 ½ pounds lean ground beef

1 yellow onion, chopped

1 red bell pepper, chopped

1 ½ cups ketchup

3 tablespoons apple cider vinegar

3 tablespoons Worcestershire sauce

3 tablespoons brown sugar

sea salt and ground black pepper to taste

3 tablespoons yellow mustard

2 tablespoons grated Parmesan cheese

5 large hamburger buns, toasted

3 tablespoons hickory flavored barbecue sauce

Directions

1

Cook the ground beef in a large skillet over medium heat until completely browned, 5 to 7 minutes. Add the onion and bell pepper, season with sea salt and black pepper, and cook until vegetables soften, about 8 minutes.

2

Stir in the ketchup, vinegar, Worcestershire sauce, brown sugar, mustard, and barbeque sauce. Reduce heat to low and simmer the mixture until thickened, about 10 minutes. Add Parmesan cheese and serve on toasted hamburger buns.

Nutritions

Per Serving: 530 calories; protein 29.6g; carbohydrates 59.4g; fat 19.5g; cholesterol 84.5mg; sodium 1531.4mg.

Beef Chuck Roast

Prep:

10 mins

Cook:

6 hrs 30 mins

Additional:

20 mins

Total:

7 hrs

Servings:

12

Yield:

12 servings

Ingredients

1 tablespoon salt
1 tablespoon garlic powder
¼ cup brown sugar
1 tablespoon Montreal steak seasoning
1 (3 pound) chuck roast, or more to taste
½ cup barbeque sauce
1 tablespoon ground black pepper

Directions

1

Preheat a smoker to 275 degrees F.

2

Combine salt, pepper, garlic powder, and steak seasoning in a bowl. Rub mixture evenly over the roast and place in a baking pan.

3

Cook roast in the smoker until meat reaches an internal temperature of 165 degrees F, 4 to 4 1/2 hours. Wrap roast in aluminum foil and continue smoking until meat reaches an internal temperature of 195 degrees F, about 1 hour more.

4

Remove roast from smoker and let sit for 20 minutes. Leave smoker on.

5

Cut meat into cubes and return to the baking dish. Add barbeque sauce and brown sugar.

6

Smoke meat for 1 1/2 to 2 hours more.

Nutritions

Per Serving: 209 calories; protein 13.4g; carbohydrates 9.4g; fat 12.8g; cholesterol 51.7mg; sodium 960.8mg.

Braised Beef Brisket

Prep:

15 mins

Cook:

2 hrs 30 mins

Total:

2 hrs 45 mins

Servings:

8

Yield:

8 servings

Ingredients

1 teaspoon dried thyme

1 teaspoon salt

1 (3 pound) beef brisket

1 tablespoon olive oil

1 red onion, sliced

¼ teaspoon ground black pepper

1 (8 ounce) can tomato sauce

½ cup red wine

1 (14.5 ounce) can beef broth

Directions

1

Preheat oven to 350 degrees F.

2

Mix thyme, salt, and black pepper in a small bowl and rub the mixture over both sides of brisket.

3

Heat olive oil in a roasting pan over medium-high heat; place brisket in the hot oil and brown on both sides, 3 to 4 minutes per side. Remove brisket from pan and set aside.

4

Place red onion slices into the hot roasting pan and cook and stir until onion is slightly softened, about 2 minutes. Stir in beef broth, tomato sauce, and wine.

5

Place the brisket back into the roasting pan and cover pan with foil.

6

Roast the brisket in the preheated oven for 1 hour; remove foil and baste brisket with pan juices. Place foil back over roasting pan and roast brisket until very tender and pan sauce has thickened, 1 1/2 to 2 more hours.

Nutritions

Per Serving: 327 calories; protein 18.4g; carbohydrates 3.3g; fat 25.1g; cholesterol 69.1mg; sodium 649mg.

Tangy Lamb Patties

Prep:

15 mins

Cook:

30 mins

Total:

45 mins

Servings:

18

Yield:

18 patties

Ingredients

1 pound ground lamb

2 tablespoons chopped fresh cilantro

5 green chile peppers, diced

1 tablespoon dark soy sauce

1 tablespoon Worcestershire sauce

2 tablespoons ginger paste

2 tablespoons garlic paste

3 onions, peeled and chopped

½ teaspoon ground white pepper

½ teaspoon ground cardamom

½ teaspoon ground cloves

½ teaspoon ground cinnamon

1 (17.5 ounce) package frozen puff pastry sheets, thawed

1 egg, beaten

Directions

1

In a large pot, combine the ground lamb, onion, chilies, soy sauce and Worcestershire sauce. Season with ginger and garlic pastes, white pepper, cinnamon, cardamom and cloves. Cook, stirring occasionally, over medium heat until the meat is evenly browned and the onions are tender, about 15 minutes. Mix in cilantro, cover and set aside.

2

Preheat the oven to 375 degrees F. Lay sheets of puff pastry out on a lightly floured surface. Cut each one into 9 squares and roll out to 1/4 inch thickness. Spoon about 1 1/2 tablespoons of the meat mixture into the center of each square. Brush the edge with water, fold corner over to form a triangle, and press to seal. Do not overstuff the triangles, or they will burst in the oven. Place the patties onto a foil lined baking sheet leaving at least an inch between each one. Brush the tops lightly with beaten egg.

3

Bake for 12 to 15 minutes in the preheated oven, or until golden brown all over. Serve hot for best flavor.

Nutritions

Per Serving: 222 calories; protein 7.2g; carbohydrates 15.7g; fat 14.1g; cholesterol 27.2mg; sodium 247mg

Sweet and Spicy Pork

Prep:

15 mins

Cook:

8 mins

Total:

23 mins

Servings:

16

Yield:

16 kabobs

Ingredients

1 Smithfield® Peppercorn & Garlic Seasoned Boneless Pork Sirloin Roast, cut into 32 (1-inch) pieces

2 large red bell peppers, cut into 16 (1-inch) pieces ·

16 (6 inch) bamboo skewers, soaked in water for 30 minutes, drained

⅔ cup honey

½ ripe pineapple, peeled, cored, and cut into 16 (1-inch) pieces

2 teaspoons Caribbean jerk seasoning blend

2 tablespoons balsamic vinegar

Directions

1

Heat broiler with rack about 8 inches from heat source.

2

Thread 2 pieces of pork, 1 pineapple cube and 1 red pepper piece onto each skewer. Wrap exposed end of each skewer with foil to discourage scorching.

3

Mix honey, vinegar and jerk seasoning together for glaze.

4

Broil kabobs, turning occasionally, until pork is done, about 8 minutes. Generously brush kabobs with honey glaze during last 2 to 3 minutes.

Nutritions

Per Serving: 174 calories; protein 6.9g; carbohydrates 15.3g; fat 9.7g; cholesterol 33mg; sodium 87.6mg.

Spanish Beef Empanadas

Prep:

45 mins

Cook:

35 mins

Total:

1 hr 20 mins

Servings:

4

Yield:

20 empanadas

Ingredients

1 tablespoon Goya Extra Virgin Olive Oil

½ pound ground beef

¼ cup Goya Tomato Sauce

6 Goya Spanish Olives Stuffed with Minced Pimientos, thinly sliced

2 tablespoons Goya Sofrito

1 packet Sazon Goya with Coriander and Annatto

½ medium yellow onion, finely chopped

1 teaspoon Goya Minced Garlic

½ teaspoon Goya Dried Oregano

1 (14 ounce) package Goya Discos (yellow or white), thawed

Goya Corn Oil, for frying

Goya Ground Black Pepper, to taste

Directions

1

Heat oil in a large skillet over medium heat. Add ground beef and cook until browned, breaking up meat with a wooden spoon, about 10 minutes. Add onions and cook until soft, about 5 minutes more. Stir in tomato sauce, olives, Sofrito, Sazon, garlic, oregano and black pepper. Lower heat to medium-low and simmer until mixture thickens, about 15 minutes.

2

On a lightly floured work surface, using a rolling pin, roll out discos until 1/2-inch larger in diameter. Spoon about 1 tbsp. meat mixture into middle, fold in half to form a half moon; moisten edges with water and pinch to seal closed, or seal with a fork.

3

Fill a deep saucepan with oil to a depth of 2 1/2-inches. Heat oil over medium-high heat until hot but not smoking (350 degrees F on deep-fry thermometer). Cook Empanadas in batches until crisp and golden brown, flipping once, 4 - 6 minutes. Transfer to paper towels to drain.

Braised Lamb Shanks

Prep:

20 mins

Cook:

3 hrs 30 mins

Total:

3 hrs 50 mins

Servings:

4

Yield:

4 servings

Ingredients

4 lamb shanks
2 tablespoons olive oil
2 teaspoons kosher salt
1 teaspoon ground cinnamon
½ teaspoon dried rosemary
1 large onion, sliced
6 cloves garlic, crushed
1 teaspoon freshly ground black pepper
1 teaspoon smoked paprika
⅓ cup saba
½ teaspoon chopped fresh rosemary
1 cup chicken broth

Directions

1

Preheat oven to 450 degrees F.

2

Place lamb shanks into a large bowl; drizzle with olive oil. Sprinkle with salt, black pepper, smoked paprika, cinnamon, and rosemary. Toss the lamb shanks to spread oil and seasonings over the meat.

3

Spread onion slices and garlic cloves into the bottom of a heavy 9x12-inch baking dish. Lay lamb shanks over onions and garlic.

4

Bake lamb in preheated oven for 30 minutes. Reduce oven temperature to 200 degrees F.

5

Combine chicken broth and saba in a bowl. Pour mixture over the lamb shanks. Cover baking dish tightly with foil and place baking dish on a baking sheet.

6

Bake lamb in the oven until a knife pierces the meat easily, 2 1/2 to 3 hours. The meat will be tender but not falling off the bone. Use tongs to turn the shanks over in the pan sauce. Increase temperature to 350 degrees F.

7

Return shanks to oven and bake, uncovered, until meat is fork-tender and the sauce has thickened slightly, 10 to 15 minutes. Turn shanks over in the sauce after 10 minutes and check for tenderness; if still not tender enough, return to oven for 10 to 15 more minutes and test again.

8

Transfer lamb shanks to a bowl and keep warm. Strain pan juices into a saucepan and place over medium heat. Bring to a boil and cook, stirring often, until thickened, about 5 minutes. Skim any excess grease from top of sauce. Taste and season with salt; stir in fresh rosemary. Serve sauce drizzled over lamb shanks.

Nutritions

Per Serving: 334 calories; protein 25.9g; carbohydrates 9.8g; fat 20.5g; cholesterol 82.4mg; sodium 1034.8mg.

Saucy Slow Cooker Pork Chops

Prep:

15 mins

Cook:

6 hrs 10 mins

Total:

6 hrs 25 mins

Servings:

5

Yield:

5 servings

Ingredients

3 tablespoons olive oil

1 (8 ounce) can tomato sauce

1 onion, sliced

2 green bell peppers, sliced

¼ cup brown sugar

1 tablespoon apple cider vinegar

2 teaspoons Worcestershire sauce

5 boneless pork chops, trimmed

1 ½ teaspoons salt

Directions

1

Heat olive oil in a large skillet over medium heat; cook pork chops in the hot oil until browned, about 5 minutes per side. Transfer browned pork chops to a slow cooker; top pork chops with onion and green peppers.

2

Whisk tomato sauce, brown sugar, vinegar, Worcestershire sauce, and salt together in a bowl. Pour sauce into slow cooker, gently stirring to coat meat and vegetables.

3

Cook pork chops on Low until tender, 6 to 8 hours.

4

Transfer pork chops to a serving platter; tent with aluminum foil to keep warm. Whisk cornstarch into sauce until thickened; spoon sauce and vegetables over pork chops.

Nutritions

Per Serving: 321 calories; protein 24.8g; carbohydrates 20.9g; fat 15.2g; cholesterol 59.1mg; sodium 994.6mg.

Beef Mini Meatloaves

Prep:

15 mins

Cook:

45 mins

Total:

1 hr

Servings:

8

Yield:

8 servings

Ingredients

1 egg

¼ cup packed brown sugar

¾ cup milk

½ cup quick cooking oats

1 teaspoon salt

1 pound ground beef

1 cup shredded Cheddar cheese

⅔ cup ketchup

1 ½ teaspoons prepared mustard

Directions

1

Preheat oven to 350 degrees F.

2

In a large bowl, combine the egg, milk, cheese, oats and salt. Add the ground beef, mixing well, and form this mixture into eight miniature meatloaves. Place these in a lightly greased 9x13 inch baking dish.

3

In a separate small bowl, combine the ketchup, brown sugar and mustard. Stir thoroughly and spread over each meatloaf.

4

Bake, uncovered, at 350 degrees F for 45 minutes.

Nutritions

Per Serving: 255 calories; protein 15.1g; carbohydrates 16.6g; fat 14.4g; cholesterol 73.9mg; sodium 656mg.

Italian Parmigiana

Prep:

30 mins

Cook:

50 mins

Additional:

8 hrs 15 mins

Total:

9 hrs 35 mins

Servings:

12

Yield:

12 servings

Ingredients

2 medium Italian eggplants, peeled and cut into 1/4-inch slices

2 cups all-purpose flour, sifted

1 tablespoon ground black pepper, or to taste

5 eggs, room temperature

3 tablespoons water, room temperature

3 tablespoons sea salt

2 cups freshly grated Pecorino-Romano cheese, divided

40 ounces Italian-style tomato sauce

2 cups freshly grated Parmesan cheese

½ cup extra-virgin olive oil

30 ounces freshly grated mozzarella cheese

Directions

1

Lay eggplant slices on top of paper towels and sprinkle with sea salt to draw out moisture. Cover with additional paper towels. Let sit, 8 hours to overnight.

2

Place flour into a 1-gallon plastic zip-top bag. Sprinkle salt and pepper into the flour and shake the bag to mix. Place 6 eggplant slices into the bag, seal, and shake to coat.

3

Beat eggs and water together using a fork in a small bowl. Season with salt and pepper.

4

Heat 2 inches of oil over medium-high heat in a 10-inch cast iron skillet. Line baking sheets with paper towels to drain eggplants after frying.

5

Shake excess flour from eggplant slices and place into egg mixture, turning to ensure both sides are coated. Allow excess egg mixture to drip off before placing slices into the hot oil. Fry until slightly golden, 2 to 3 minutes per side. Transfer to the paper towel-lined baking sheets. Sprinkle with 1 tablespoon Pecorino Romano cheese. Repeat process until all eggplant slices are fried. Let cool slightly, about 5 minutes.

6

Preheat the oven to 375 degrees F.

7

Pour a small amount of tomato sauce into the bottom of a 9x13-inch baking pan to cover. Place 1/3 of the eggplant slices over sauce, slightly overlapping them. Sprinkle 1/3 of the remaining Pecorino-Romano cheese and Parmesan cheese evenly over the slices. Cover with a light layer of sauce. Sprinkle 1/3 of the mozzarella cheese over sauce. Repeat for a total of 3 layers.

8

Bake in the preheated oven until bubbly, about 40 minutes. Remove from the oven and let cool for 10 minutes to set.

Nutritions

Per Serving: 569 calories; protein 35.6g; carbohydrates 33.1g; fat 32.7g; cholesterol 145.9mg; sodium 2463.2mg.

Pork Stew

Prep:

15 mins

Cook:

2 hrs

Total:

2 hrs 15 mins

Servings:

4

Yield:

4 servings

Ingredients

2 ½ pounds pork shoulder, cut into 2-inch chunks

¼ cup chicken broth

salt and freshly ground black pepper to taste

2 tablespoons vegetable oil

1 large yellow onion, chopped

2 tablespoons apple cider vinegar

½ cup apple cider or apple juice

2 tablespoons Dijon mustard

1 tablespoon prepared horseradish

3 cloves minced garlic

1 ¼ cups heavy cream

1 stalk celery, sliced

1 cup sliced carrots

4 sage leaves

2 sprigs thyme

1 dried bay leaf

2 small sprigs fresh rosemary

1 pinch cayenne pepper

½ cup green peas, fresh or frozen

¼ cup matchstick-cut apple strips

1 tablespoon chopped fresh chives

Directions

1

Season pork chunks generously with salt and pepper. Toss to distribute seasonings evenly.

2

Heat vegetable oil in pot over high heat. Brown pork in batches so meat isn't crowded, about 7 minutes total time per batch. Transfer pork to a plate. Cook onions in same pot; cook and stir until they start to turn translucent and edges get brown, 3 or 4 minutes. Add garlic; cook 1 minute. Stir in apple cider and apple cider vinegar.

3

Raise heat to high. Stir in mustard and horseradish. Transfer browned pork pieces back to pot, along with accumulated juices. Pour in cream and chicken broth to cover. Add sage, thyme, rosemary, and bay leaf. Season with a pinch of salt. Bring to a simmer; reduce heat, cover, and simmer on low for 30 minutes. Add celery, carrots, black pepper and cayenne.

4

Simmer uncovered on low until meat is tender, about 1 hour. Add green peas. Simmer another 10 minutes. Optional: for a thicker sauce, raise heat and simmer until sauce is reduced, 6 to 8 minutes.

5

Garnish individual servings with apple strips and chopped fresh chives.

Nutritions

Per Serving: 760 calories; protein 32.5g; carbohydrates 19.6g; fat 61.2g; cholesterol 213.8mg; sodium 446.5mg.

Tender Pork Stew with Beans

Prep:

20 mins

Cook:

1 hr 50 mins

Total:

2 hrs 10 mins

Servings:

8

Yield:

8 servings

Ingredients

2 ½ (2 pound) pork tenderloin, trimmed and sliced1 1/2-inch thick

1 tablespoon olive oil

2 onions, diced

2 red bell peppers, diced

2 tablespoons minced garlic

3 (14.5 ounce) cans diced tomatoes with green chile peppers

2 (15 ounce) cans kidney beans, rinsed and drained

1 ½ cups beef broth

salt and ground black pepper to taste

1 teaspoon dried basil

1 teaspoon ground cumin

1 (9 ounce) bag frozen shelled edamame

2 teaspoons chili powder

1 (4 ounce) can diced green chile peppers

Directions

1

Season pork tenderloin with salt and black pepper.

2

Heat olive oil in a large Dutch oven or heavy pot over medium-high heat. Add pork to hot oil and cook until browned, 1 to 2 minutes per side. Add onions, red bell peppers, and garlic to pork; cook and stir until onion is slightly tender, about 10 minutes.

3

Stir tomatoes with green chile peppers, kidney beans, beef broth, green chile peppers, chili powder, basil, and cumin into pork mixture. Bring mixture to a boil, reduce heat to medium-low, cover Dutch oven, and simmer, stirring every 15 minutes, until pork is tender and falling apart, 1 1/2 to 2 hours.

4

Stir edamame, corn, and carrots into stew; cook until heated through, about 5 minutes. Break pork into pieces using the flat edge of a wooden spoon creating a 'shredded' texture.

Nutritions

Per Serving: 581 calories; protein 72g; carbohydrates 39.6g; fat 15.1g; cholesterol 184.4mg; sodium 1330.8mg.

Barbecue Pork

Prep:

20 mins

Cook:

40 mins

Additional:

4 hrs

Total:

5 hrs

Servings:

4

Yield:

4 servings

Ingredients

1 (2 pound) pork shoulder

¼ cup grated onion

1 tablespoon light brown sugar

2 teaspoons kosher salt

1 teaspoon freshly ground black pepper

1 teaspoon paprika

1 large clove garlic, finely grated

¼ teaspoon cayenne pepper

½ cup prepared barbecue sauce

½ teaspoon ground cumin

Directions

1

Slice the pork shoulder in half lengthwise. Cut each piece across into thin, 1/8-inch slices.

2

Transfer pork to a mixing bowl and add garlic, onion, brown sugar, salt, pepper, paprika, cumin, and cayenne. Mix with your hands until thoroughly combined.

3

Wrap in plastic wrap and transfer into a refrigerator for 4 hours, or up to overnight.

4

Preheat an charcoal grill for medium-high heat and lightly oil the grate.

5

Weave pork slices on metal skewers, folding the longer pieces in half as you go. Slices should be pressed snugly together as you build the skewer.

6

Grill skewers over the hot charcoal until browned and no longer pink, turning frequently, about 30 minutes. Brush on barbecue sauce and turn skewers several times so the sauce caramelizes, about 10 minutes more. An instant-read thermometer inserted into the center should read at least 160 degrees F. Serve immediately.

Nutritions

Per Serving: 359 calories; protein 23.4g; carbohydrates 16.9g; fat 21.5g; cholesterol 89.1mg; sodium 1379.5mg.

Chicken Tacos

Servings:

4

Yield:

8 tacos

Ingredients

1 cup barbecue sauce

1 tablespoon Southwest seasoning

2 teaspoons olive oil

3 cups shredded rotisserie chicken

8 (6 inch) flour or corn tortillas

½ teaspoon hot sauce

½ cup chopped tomatoes

½ cup coarsely chopped fresh cilantro

Lime wedges, for serving

½ cup Borden® Finely Shredded Four Cheese Mexican Shreds

Directions

1

Combine barbecue sauce, seasoning and hot sauce in a small bowl. Let stand 15 minutes.

2

Heat oil in a large skillet over medium heat until hot.

3

Add chicken; cook and stir 3 to 5 minutes or until warmed through.

4

Add barbecue sauce mixture. Cook 3 to 5 minutes more or until chicken is coated and sauce thickens slightly.

5

Heat tortillas according to package directions.

6

Spoon chicken mixture evenly onto the center of each tortilla.

7

Top each taco evenly with tomatoes, Borden® Queso Fresco Fresh Crumbling Cheese and cilantro. Serve with lime wedges.

Nutritions

Per Serving: 626 calories; protein 37.3g; carbohydrates 57.6g; fat 26.4g; cholesterol 107.4mg; sodium 1456.7mg.

Turkey Kebabs

Prep:

45 mins

Cook:

5 mins

Additional:

30 mins

Total:

1 hr 20 mins

Servings:

28

Yield:

28 skewers

Ingredients

4 cloves garlic, minced

¼ teaspoon cayenne pepper

1 teaspoon kosher salt

1 pound ground lamb

3 tablespoons chopped fresh parsley

1 tablespoon ground coriander

1 teaspoon ground cumin

½ tablespoon ground cinnamon

3 tablespoons grated onion

½ teaspoon ground allspice

¼ teaspoon ground ginger

¼ teaspoon ground black pepper

28 bamboo skewers, soaked in water for 30 minutes

Directions

1

Mash the garlic into a paste with the salt using a mortar and pestle or the flat side of a chef's knife on your cutting board. Mix the garlic into the lamb along with the onion, parsley, coriander, cumin, cinnamon, allspice, cayenne pepper, ginger, and pepper in a mixing bowl until well blended. Form the mixture into 28 balls. Form each ball around the tip of a skewer, flattening into a 2 inch oval; repeat with the remaining skewers. Place the kebabs onto a baking sheet, cover, and refrigerate at least 30 minutes, or up to 12 hours.

2

Preheat an outdoor grill for medium heat, and lightly oil grate.

3

Cook the skewers on the preheated grill, turning occasionally, until the lamb has cooked to your desired degree of doneness, about 6 minutes for medium.

Nutritions

Per Serving: 35 calories; protein 2.9g; carbohydrates 0.6g; fat 2.3g; cholesterol 10.8mg; sodium 78.2mg.

Pork Tenderloin

Prep:

5 mins

Cook:

20 mins

Additional:

5 mins

Total:

30 mins

Servings:

12

Yield:

12 servings

Ingredients

4 pounds pork tenderloin

4 teaspoons garlic, minced

2 teaspoons dried oregano

1 teaspoon salt

1 teaspoon ground black pepper

2 teaspoons dried rosemary

Directions

1

Preheat the oven to 425 degrees F.

2

Combine garlic, rosemary, oregano, salt, and pepper in a small bowl. Rub spice mixture all over the pork tenderloin. Place in a baking dish.

3

Bake in the preheated oven until pork is slightly pink in the center, 20 to 25 minutes. An instant-read thermometer inserted into the center should read at least 145 degrees F. Remove from oven and let stand for 5 minutes before slicing.

Nutritions

Per Serving: 183 calories; protein 26.9g; carbohydrates 0.7g; fat 7.3g; cholesterol 84.2mg; sodium 251.5mg.

Pork and Vegetable Souvlaki

Prep:

10 mins

Cook:

15 mins

Additional:

1 day

Total:

1 day

Servings:

8

Yield:

8 servings

Ingredients

2 pounds pork tenderloin, cut into 1 1/2-inch cubes

3 bay leaves, broken into pieces

½ cup olive oil

½ cup dry white wine

1 lemon, juiced

2 teaspoons dried oregano

salt and ground black pepper to taste

2 cloves garlic, chopped

Directions

1

Place pork tenderloin cubes into a gallon-sized resealable bag.

2

Stir olive oil, dry white wine, lemon juice, garlic, oregano, salt, and pepper together in a bowl. Pour over pork in the bag and mix well.

3

Let pork marinate in the refrigerator for at least 1 day, up to 5 days.

4

Remove pork cubes from marinade and thread onto metal skewers. Place bay leaf pieces between meat cubes.

5

Preheat an outdoor grill for medium heat and lightly oil the grate.

6

Arrange skewers on the preheated grill. Turn the kabobs and baste with marinade frequently for the first 10 minutes of cooking, then discard marinade. Cook about 6 minutes longer, until pork is cooked through and juices run clear.

Nutritions

Per Serving: 233 calories; protein 17.8g; carbohydrates 2.4g; fat 15.9g; cholesterol 49mg; sodium 59.3mg.

Maiale al Latte

Prep:

15 mins

Cook:

1 hr 35 mins

Total:

1 hr 50 mins

Servings:

4

Yield:

4 servings

Ingredients

1 tablespoon olive oil

2 slices bacon, coarsely chopped

salt and freshly ground black pepper to taste

1 small yellow onion, diced

4 cloves garlic, sliced

1 ¼ cups chicken broth

½ cup creme fraiche

1 ½ pounds pork shoulder, cut into 2-inch chunks

2 tablespoons chopped fresh sage leaves

¼ cup olive oil

15 whole fresh sage leaves

1 pinch red pepper flakes

Directions

1

Pour 1 tablespoon olive oil into a skillet, place over medium heat, and cook bacon, stirring often, until crisp and bacon fat has rendered into the skillet, about 5 minutes.

2

Season pork cubes generously with salt and black pepper. Remove bacon from pan and set aside, reserving fat in pan. Turn heat to medium-high and brown pork pieces in bacon drippings until well browned on both sides, about 5 minutes per side. Transfer meat to a bowl, leaving pan drippings in skillet.

3

Turn heat to medium and stir in chopped onion and a pinch of salt. Cook and stir onion until translucent and slightly browned, about 5 minutes. Stir garlic into onion and cook until fragrant, about 1 minute.

4

Pour chicken broth and creme fraiche into onion mixture; whisk until smooth. Scrape up and dissolve any browned bits of food on the bottom of the skillet. Bring mixture to a simmer.

5

Return bacon to sauce and stir in 2 tablespoons chopped sage. Place pork pieces into simmering sauce along with any accumulated juices from the meat. Reduce heat to low, cover, and simmer until meat is almost tender, about 1 hour.

6

Raise heat to medium and cook uncovered until pan sauce reduces and thickens and meat is very tender, about 20 more minutes. Stir red pepper flakes into sauce; adjust seasonings to taste.

7

Heat 1/4 cup olive oil in a small skillet over medium heat; drop whole sage leaves into the hot oil and cook, lightly tossing leaves in the oil, until crisp, about 15 seconds. Drain sage leaves on paper towels and crumble over pork.

Nutritions

Per Serving: 514 calories; protein 20.9g; carbohydrates 4.7g; fat 46.2g; cholesterol 114.4mg; sodium 568.8mg.

Apricot-Glazed Pork Ribs

Prep:

10 mins

Cook:

1 hr 40 mins

Additional:

8 hrs

Total:

9 hrs 50 mins

Servings:

12

Yield:

12 servings

Ingredients

3 ½ pounds baby back pork ribs
salt and ground black pepper to taste
⅓ cup soy sauce
¼ cup packed light brown sugar
2 teaspoons garlic powder
1 (16 ounce) jar apricot preserves
aluminum foil

Directions

1

Place ribs in a large roasting pan. Whisk together apricot preserves, soy sauce, brown sugar, and garlic powder until blended. Pour apricot marinade over ribs, cover, and place in the refrigerator, 8 hours to overnight.

2

Preheat the oven to 325 degrees F. Line a baking pan with aluminum foil.

3

Remove ribs from the marinade and shake off excess. Place ribs in the prepared baking pan and season with salt and pepper. Pour marinade into a small saucepan and bring to a boil. Reduce heat and simmer marinade for 5 minutes; set aside.

4

Bake ribs in the preheated oven, basting frequently with the cooked marinade, until ribs are tender and meat pulls away easily from the bone, about 1 hour 30 minutes. An instant-read thermometer inserted into the center should read 145 degrees F.

Nutritions

Per Serving: 327 calories; protein 14.8g; carbohydrates 29.4g; fat 17.2g; cholesterol 68.2mg; sodium 488.5mg.

Pan-Fried Chive Flowers

Prep:

10 mins

Cook:

5 mins

Total:

15 mins

Servings:

2

Yield:

2 servings

Ingredients

1 tablespoon olive oil

1 ½ cups fresh chive flowers, rinsed and well-drained

1 clove garlic, minced

salt

black pepper

1 tablespoon butter

Directions

1

Heat olive oil in a large skillet over medium-high heat. Add butter; heat until melted, about 30 seconds. Add chive flowers, garlic, and salt; cook and stir until soft and tender, 3 to 5 minutes. Grind black pepper over mixture before serving.

Nutritions

Per Serving: 125 calories; protein 1.4g; carbohydrates 2.4g; fat 12.8g; cholesterol 15.3mg; sodium 120.1mg.

Oven-Roasted Spare Ribs

Prep:

15 mins

Cook:

2 hrs 20 mins

Total:

2 hrs 35 mins

Servings:

4

Yield:

4 servings

Ingredients

1 teaspoon vegetable oil

½ teaspoon dry mustard

½ cup chopped onions

¾ cup chili sauce

½ cup beer

¼ cup honey

2 cloves minced garlic

3 ½ pounds country style pork ribs

2 tablespoons Worcestershire sauce

Directions

1

Heat oil in a saucepan over medium-high heat. Cook and stir onions and garlic in hot oil until fragrant and softened, 4 to 6 minutes.

2

Stir chili sauce, beer, honey, Worcestershire sauce, and dry mustard into onion mixture; bring to a boil, reduce heat to low, and simmer until sauce thickens and flavors develop, 20 minutes.

3

Preheat oven to 350 degrees F.

4

Bake ribs in a baking dish in the preheated oven for 1 hour. Spread sauce over ribs and return to oven; bake until sauce bubbles and ribs are tender, 1 hour.

Nutritions

Per Serving: 634 calories; protein 47.9g; carbohydrates 35.5g; fat 32.2g; cholesterol 178.7mg; sodium 871.5mg.

Duck Breasts with Raspberry Sauce

Prep:

20 mins

Cook:

30 mins

Total:

50 mins

Servings:

4

Yield:

4 servings

Ingredients

4 duck breast halves

2 teaspoons ground cinnamon

1 teaspoon cornstarch

4 teaspoons demerara sugar

½ cup red wine

¼ cup creme de cassis liqueur

2 teaspoons sea salt

4 ounces raspberries

Directions

1

Preheat oven on broiler setting. Use a fork to score the duck breasts through the skin and fat but not all the way through to the meat.

2

Heat a large heavy skillet on medium high. Fry the duck breasts skin side down, until the skin browns and fat runs out, about 10 minutes. Remove the breasts from the pan, and pour off most of the fat. Return breasts to pan, and fry skin side up for another 10 minutes. Remove breasts from pan, and allow to rest on a baking sheet. Mix the sea salt, cinnamon and Demerara sugar together and sprinkle over the skin of the duck breasts. Pour most of the fat out of the frying pan.

3

Mix together the red wine, cassis, and cornstarch in a small bowl. Pour into the pan, and simmer for 3 minutes, stirring constantly, until the sauce is thickened. Add raspberries, and simmer for another minute until heated through.

4

Broil the duck breasts skin side up, until the sugar begins to caramelize, about 1 minute. Slice the duck breasts thinly, pour a little sauce over the top, and serve warm.

Nutritions

Per Serving: 395 calories; protein 45.3g; carbohydrates 15.2g; fat 9.9g; cholesterol 174.6mg; sodium 1011.8mg.

Salt and Pepper Spare Ribs

Prep:

10 mins

Cook:

3 hrs

Additional:

4 hrs 15 mins

Total:

7 hrs 25 mins

Servings:

8

Yield:

8 servings

Ingredients

4 teaspoons kosher salt

1 tablespoon freshly ground black pepper

1 teaspoon cayenne pepper

½ teaspoon garlic powder

1 rack St. Louis-style pork spare ribs

2 teaspoons Dijon mustard

2 tablespoons white vinegar

1 teaspoon freshly ground white pepper

Directions

1

Mix salt, black pepper, white pepper, cayenne, and garlic powder together in a small bowl. Set spice rub aside.

2

Stir Dijon mustard and vinegar together in a small bowl.

3

Place ribs on a foil-lined baking sheet. Turn the ribs over so that the meat side is down. Use the tip of a small, sharp knife to make some very shallow slashes every few inches through the membrane that covers the ribs. Poke the knife 3 or 4 times between each rib bone, about 1/4 inch deep.

4

Brush about 1/2 of the Dijon mustard mixture on top. Sprinkle with about 40% of the spice rub. Turn the rack over and brush on the rest of the mustard and vinegar mixture. Sprinkle on the rest of the rub, reserving 1 or 2 teaspoons in case you want to use it to season the cooked ribs later.

5

Refrigerate the ribs, uncovered, 4 to 12 hours before baking.

6

Preheat the oven to 300 degrees F. Remove ribs from the refrigerator.

7

Cook in the center of the preheated oven for 1 1/2 hours. Remove from the oven and baste with the pan drippings. Continue to cook until very tender and the tip of a knife slides in very easily, about 1 1/2 hours more.

8

Remove from the oven, baste again, and let ribs rest for 15 minutes before cutting and serving.

Nutritions

Per Serving: 400 calories; protein 29.1g; carbohydrates 1.2g; fat 30.2g; cholesterol 120.2mg; sodium 1084.1mg.

Keto Bacon-Wrapped Asparagus with Lemon Aioli

Prep:

15 mins

Cook:

20 mins

Total:

35 mins

Servings:

5

Yield:

5 servings

Ingredients

Lemon Aioli:

1 teaspoon Dijon mustard

¾ cup mayonnaise

1 clove garlic, minced

1 tablespoon fresh lemon juice

¼ teaspoon garlic salt

1 teaspoon lemon zest

Asparagus Bundles:

1 bunch fresh asparagus, trimmed

olive oil cooking spray

1 pinch cracked black pepper

10 slices bacon

Directions

1

Combine mayonnaise, Dijon mustard, garlic, lemon zest, lemon juice, and garlic salt in a bowl and mix well. Refrigerate lemon aioli until ready to use.

2

Preheat an outdoor grill for medium heat and lightly oil the grate.

3

Divide asparagus stalks into groups of 3 to 5 stalks, depending on the thickness of the asparagus. Wrap each asparagus bundle tightly with 1 piece of bacon, overlapping slightly as you wrap and tucking the ends under the bacon so it holds securely.

4

Place asparagus bundles in a single layer on a piece of aluminum foil. Spray bundles lightly with olive oil spray and top the bacon with cracked pepper.

5

Grill asparagus bundles on the foil for 10 minutes. Flip each bundle and grill until bacon is cooked through and crisp, an additional 10 minutes. Serve with lemon aioli.

Nutritions

Per Serving: 359 calories; protein 9.2g; carbohydrates 5.7g; fat 34.1g; cholesterol 32.8mg; sodium 730.1mg.

Mississipi Pulled Pork

Prep:

10 mins

Cook:

8 hrs 30 mins

Total:

8 hrs 40 mins

Servings:

12

Yield:

12 servings

Ingredients

1 tablespoon barbeque spice rub

1 (18 ounce) bottle barbecue sauce

1 (3 pound) boneless pork loin roast

Directions

1

Preheat the oven to 225 degrees F. Place a small rack inside a Dutch oven.

2

Rub pork roast with barbecue spice rub and place on the rack in the prepared Dutch oven.

3

Cover and cook in the preheated oven until roast is fork-tender, about 8 hours.

4

Shred the roast with 2 forks and return meat to the Dutch oven with some of the roasting juices and a generous amount of barbeque sauce.

5

Let simmer over medium heat for at least 30 minutes.

Nutritions

Per Serving: 160 calories; protein 13.2g; carbohydrates 15.5g; fat 4.5g; cholesterol 39.8mg; sodium 722.3mg.

Chicken Liver Pate

Prep:

20 mins

Cook:

15 mins

Additional:

3 hrs 30 mins

Total:

4 hrs 5 mins

Servings:

16

Yield:

2 cups

Ingredients

1 cup butter, divided

¼ teaspoon ground black pepper

1 onion, quartered

1 pound chicken livers, rinsed and trimmed

¼ cup brandy

2 tablespoons heavy whipping cream

1 teaspoon lemon juice

1 tart apple - peeled, cored, and quartered

1 ½ teaspoons salt

1 tablespoon butter, melted

Directions

1

Set aside 1/2 cup butter to soften slightly.

2

Place onion and apple in a food processor with the steel knife blade; process until coarsely chopped.

3

Melt 3 tablespoons butter in a large skillet over medium heat. Add onion and apple; cook and stir until lightly browned, 5 to 10 minutes. Return onion and apple to food processor.

4

Melt 5 tablespoons butter in the same skillet over high heat; cook chicken livers until browned and just done inside, about 5 minutes. Reduce heat to low and pour in brandy; allow to warm up without stirring. Carefully light the liquid; let flames subside.

5

Transfer chicken liver mixture to the food processor with onion and apple. Add cream and process until very smooth. Transfer mixture into a bowl and refrigerate until cool, at least 30 minutes.

6

Cut the softened 1/2 cup butter into pieces and process in the food processor; add about 1/3 of the liver mixture and blend about 5 seconds. Repeat 2 more times with remaining liver mixture. Add lemon juice, salt, and pepper and blend well.

7

Transfer pate to a serving dish or several small dishes; top with 1 tablespoon melted butter. Cover loosely with plastic wrap; refrigerate until chilled and set, about 3 hours.

Nutritions

Per Serving: 165 calories; protein 4.8g; carbohydrates 2.7g; fat 14.1g; cholesterol 137.4mg; sodium 320.1mg.

Mini Pumpkin Butterscotch Muffins

Prep:

15 mins

Cook:

10 mins

Total:

25 mins

Servings:

48

Yield:

48 muffins

Ingredients

1 ¾ cups all-purpose flour

½ cup white sugar

1 teaspoon ground cinnamon

½ teaspoon ground ginger

½ teaspoon ground nutmeg

½ cup brown sugar

1 teaspoon baking soda

½ teaspoon salt

½ cup melted butter

¼ teaspoon baking powder

1 cup canned pumpkin

1 (6 ounce) package butterscotch chips

2 eggs

Directions

1

Preheat oven to 350 degrees F. Grease mini-muffin pan with cooking spray.

2

Sift together the flour, brown sugar, white sugar, cinnamon, ginger, nutmeg, baking soda, baking powder, and salt into a large bowl. Whisk together the eggs, butter, and pumpkin in a separate bowl. Mix the flour mixture with the egg mixture. Stir in the butterscotch chips; pour into each cup of the muffin pan to about 3/4 full.

3

Bake in preheated oven until a toothpick inserted into the center of a muffin comes out clean, 10 to 12 minutes.

Nutritions

Per Serving: 75 calories; protein 0.8g; carbohydrates 10.5g; fat 3.2g; cholesterol 12.8mg; sodium 86.3mg.

Vegetable Casserole with Eggplant

Prep:

20 mins

Cook:

50 mins

Total:

1 hr 10 mins

Servings:

6

Yield:

6 servings

Ingredients

1 large eggplant, peeled and diced

3 tablespoons butter

6 ounces grated sharp Cheddar cheese

3 tablespoons flour

1 green bell pepper, chopped

1 medium onion, chopped

2 tablespoons brown sugar, or more to taste

1 teaspoon salt

1 (28 ounce) can stewed tomatoes

⅓ cup fine bread crumbs

Directions

1

Preheat the oven to 350 degrees F.

2

Bring a large saucepan of water to a boil. Add eggplant and cook until tender, 10 to 15 minutes. Drain and pour eggplant into an 8-inch square baking dish.

3

Melt butter in a 3-quart saucepan on medium heat. Add flour and mix to create a paste. Add tomatoes, bell pepper, onion, brown sugar, and salt and cook over medium to medium-high heat. Stir occasionally until mixture bubbles and thickens, 5 to 10 minutes. Pour mixture over the eggplant in the baking dish.

4

Cover the vegetables in the baking dish with Cheddar cheese and bread crumbs.

5

Bake in the preheated oven until hot and bubbly, 30 to 40 minutes.

Nutritions

Per Serving: 281 calories; protein 10.9g; carbohydrates 26.4g; fat 15.9g; cholesterol 45mg; sodium 840.2mg.

Halibut Steaks with Corn and Chanterelles

Prep:

20 mins

Cook:

20 mins

Total:

40 mins

Servings:

2

Yield:

2 servings

Ingredients

2 large halibut steaks
salt and ground black pepper to taste
2 tablespoons olive oil
1 cup corn kernels
⅓ cup diced roasted red peppers
½ cup water
2 cups sliced chanterelle mushrooms
1 tablespoon butter
1 tablespoon minced fresh tarragon
1 lemon, juiced

Directions

1

Preheat grill for medium-high heat and lightly oil the grate. Season halibut steaks with salt and black pepper.

2

Heat olive oil in a skillet over medium heat. Cook and stir chanterelle mushrooms with a pinch of salt in hot oil until soft and caramelized, about 10 minutes. Stir corn and peppers into mushrooms until corn is toasted, about 2 minutes.

3

Pour water into mushroom mixture; bring to a simmer and cook until reduced, about 5 minutes. Stir lemon juice and butter into mushroom mixture until butter melts and liquid is almost evaporated.

4

Cook halibut steaks on the preheated grill until until the fish flakes easily with a fork, 3 to 5 minutes per side. Divide mushroom mixture between two plates and sprinkle tarragon over each. Top mushrooms with halibut steaks.

Nutritions

Per Serving: 562 calories; protein 53.6g; carbohydrates 30.9g; fat 25.7g; cholesterol 86.8mg; sodium 339.1mg.

Prawns with a rich tomato sauce

Prep:

15 mins

Cook:

1 hr 40 mins

Total:

1 hr 55 mins

Servings:

6

Yield:

6 servings

Ingredients

1 cup butter, divided
1 (28 ounce) can crushed tomatoes
2 pounds large prawns - peeled, deveined and butterflied
1 medium head garlic, peeled and minced
1 medium head garlic, peeled and minced
¼ cup chopped fresh parsley

Directions

1

Melt 1/2 cup butter in a saucepan over low heat. Add 1 minced head of garlic and saute for 2 to 3 minutes until soft. Stir in the tomatoes and bring to a simmer. Continue cooking until reduced to a thick paste, about 60 to 90 minutes.

2

In a separate saucepan, melt remaining 1/2 cup butter in a saucepan over low heat. Saute remaining garlic for 2 to 3 minutes.

3

Toss prawns in garlic butter sauce and place on a baking sheet. Broil until pink, do not overcook.

4

Spread the warm tomato mixture onto serving plates. Place prawns on top of tomato sauce and sprinkle with chopped parsley.

Nutritions

Per Serving: 523 calories; protein 33.1g; carbohydrates 24g; fat 33.7g; cholesterol 81.3mg; sodium 395mg.

Carrot Casserole

Prep:

15 mins

Cook:

30 mins

Total:

45 mins

Servings:

6

Yield:

6 servings

Ingredients

5 cups sliced carrots

3 tablespoons butter

1 onion, chopped

1 (10.75 ounce) can condensed cream of celery soup

salt and pepper to taste

½ cup cubed processed cheese

2 cups seasoned croutons

⅓ cup melted butter

Directions

1

Preheat oven to 350 degrees F. Grease a 2 quart casserole dish.

2

Bring a pot of water to a boil. Add carrots and cook until tender but still firm, about 8 minutes; drain.

3

Melt 3 tablespoons butter in a medium saucepan. Saute onions and stir in soup, salt, pepper and cheese. Stir in cooked carrots. Transfer mixture to prepared dish.

4

Toss croutons with 1/3 cup melted butter; scatter over casserole.

5

Bake in preheated oven for 20 to 30 minutes, or until heated through.

Nutritions

Per Serving: 331 calories; protein 6g; carbohydrates 23.1g; fat 24.6g; cholesterol 60.7mg; sodium 909.3mg.

Zingy Pesto Tuna Wrap

Prep:

15 mins

Total:

15 mins

Servings:

1

Yield:

1 wrap

Ingredients

1 (5 ounce) can albacore tuna in water, drained and flaked

2 tablespoons mayonnaise

1 teaspoon lemon juice

1 slice provolone cheese

1 pinch ground black pepper

1 (10 inch) flour tortilla

4 leaves lettuce

1 tablespoon basil pesto sauce

5 pitted kalamata olives, cut in half

Directions

1

Lightly stir together the tuna, mayonnaise, pesto, lemon juice, and pepper in a bowl until well combined.

2

Microwave the tortilla on High until warmed and pliable, 5 to 10 seconds.

3

Spread the tuna mixture on the tortilla, and top with the lettuce leaves, provolone cheese, and kalamata olives. Fold the bottom of the tortilla up about 2 inches to enclose the filling, and roll the tortilla tightly into a compact wrap.

Nutritions

Per Serving: 834 calories; protein 49.9g; carbohydrates 42.3g; fat 51.2g; cholesterol 93.8mg; sodium 1806.4mg.

Tarte Flambee

Prep:

20 mins

Cook:

20 mins

Total:

40 mins

Servings:

4

Yield:

4 servings

Ingredients

2 tablespoons butter

½ cup creme fraiche

2 onions, sliced

1 cup mushrooms, sliced

salt and ground black pepper to taste

1 (11 ounce) package thin-crust pizza dough, at room temperature

8 strips cooked bacon

½ cup fromage blanc (French-style fresh cheese)

Directions

1

Preheat oven to 400 degrees F. Lightly grease a baking sheet.

2

Melt butter in a large skillet over medium heat. Add onions and mushrooms; cook and stir until tender, about 5 minutes. Remove from heat and let cool slightly.

3

Combine creme fraiche and fromage blanc in a small bowl. Season with salt and pepper.

4

Spread pizza dough onto the prepared baking sheet. Spoon creme fraiche mixture on top. Cover evenly with onions, mushrooms, and bacon strips, leaving a 1-inch border. Scatter mozzarella cheese on top.

5

Bake in the preheated oven until crust is deep golden brown, about 15 minutes.

Nutritions

Per Serving: 476 calories; protein 15.3g; carbohydrates 49.6g; fat 24.4g; cholesterol 73.5mg; sodium 701.3mg.

Spicy Fish Curry

Prep:

15 mins

Cook:

25 mins

Additional:

10 mins

Total:

50 mins

Servings:

6

Yield:

6 servings

Ingredients

2 pounds white carp, cut into large chunks

1 tablespoon chopped fresh coriander (cilantro)

1 tablespoon vegetable oil

1 tablespoon red chile powder

1 ½ teaspoons salt

¼ cup tamarind pulp

1 cup warm water

1 tablespoon ground turmeric

¼ cup oil

½ teaspoon cumin seeds

1 ½ tablespoons garlic paste

2 tablespoons red chile powder

2 tablespoons ground coriander

1 pinch salt to taste

1 large onion, minced

Directions

1

Place fish in a bowl; add 1 tablespoon vegetable oil, 1 tablespoon chile powder, turmeric, and 1 1/2 teaspoons salt and allow to marinate for about 10 minutes.

2

Place tamarind pulp in a bowl and pour warm water over it. Squeeze tamarind to extract juice.

3

Heat 1/4 cup oil in a skillet over medium heat; add cumin seeds and stir. Add onion to cumin; cook and stir until onion is translucent, 5 to 10 minutes. Add garlic paste and cook for 3 minutes. Add carp, cover the skillet, and cook for 5 minutes.

4

Mix tamarind juice into fish mixture; bring to a boil. Turn carp pieces; add 2 tablespoons red chile powder, coriander, and salt. Cook over low heat until sauce thickens and oil separates, about 10 minutes. Garnish with coriander leaves.

Nutritions

Per Serving: 360 calories; protein 28.4g; carbohydrates 12.5g; fat 21.1g; cholesterol 99.3mg; sodium 855.6mg.

Oven-Baked Fillets

Prep:

10 mins

Cook:

20 mins

Total:

30 mins

Servings:

6

Yield:

6 servings

Ingredients

1 tablespoon vegetable oil

¼ cup butter, melted

2 pounds mackerel fillets

1 teaspoon salt

2 tablespoons lemon juice

⅛ teaspoon ground paprika

⅛ teaspoon ground black pepper

Directions

1

Preheat oven to 350 degrees F. Grease a baking pan with vegetable oil.

2

Place mackerel fillets in the baking pan; season with salt and pepper.

3

Mix butter, lemon juice, and paprika together in a bowl. Pour over mackerel fillets.

4

Bake in the preheated oven until mackerel flakes easily with a fork, 20 to 25 minutes.

Nutritions

Per Serving: 399 calories; protein 28.3g; carbohydrates 0.5g; fat 31g; cholesterol 109mg; sodium 540.2mg.

Stuffed Tomatoes

Prep:

15 mins

Cook:

45 mins

Additional:

15 mins

Total:

1 hr 15 mins

Servings:

8

Yield:

8 servings

Ingredients

½ cup dry grits

1 ½ cups water

¾ teaspoon salt

1 ⅓ cups ricotta cheese

⅓ cup grated Parmesan cheese

½ cup grated Asiago cheese

2 eggs

cooking spray

2 ½ teaspoons garlic powder

¼ teaspoon crushed red pepper

1 teaspoon salt

8 tomatoes

¼ cup chopped fresh parsley

Directions

1

In a small pot combine dry grits, 1 1/2 cups water, and 3/4 teaspoon of salt. Bring to a boil, then simmer until grits are tender, 16 to 20 minutes. Cool.

2

Preheat an oven to 350 degrees F. Coat a baking sheet with nonstick cooking spray.

3

Beat the eggs in a large bowl, then stir in the cooled grits, ricotta cheese, Parmesan cheese, and Asiago cheese. Stir in the garlic powder, parsley, crushed red pepper, and 1 teaspoon salt. Mix well.

4

Slice the top off of each tomato. Use a spoon to hollow out the tomatoes, leaving the outer shells (approximately 1/4 inch thick) intact. Fill each with the grits mixture. Arrange stuffed tomatoes on prepared baking sheet.

5

Bake in preheated oven until light golden brown, 30 to 40 minutes. Allow to cool slightly before serving.

Nutritions

Per Serving: 123 calories; protein 6.9g; carbohydrates 14.6g; fat 4.6g; cholesterol 55.5mg; sodium 669.7mg.

Baked Haddock

Prep:

10 mins

Cook:

15 mins

Total:

25 mins

Servings:

4

Yield:

4 servings

Ingredients

¾ cup milk

2 teaspoons salt

¾ cup bread crumbs

¼ teaspoon ground dried thyme

4 haddock fillets

¼ cup butter, melted

¼ cup grated Parmesan cheese

Directions

1

Preheat oven to 500 degrees F.

2

In a small bowl, combine the milk and salt. In a separate bowl, mix together the bread crumbs, Parmesan cheese, and thyme. Dip the haddock fillets in the milk, then press into the crumb mixture to coat.

Place haddock fillets in a glass baking dish, and drizzle with melted butter.

3

Bake on the top rack of the preheated oven until the fish flakes easily, about 15 minutes.

Nutritions

Per Serving: 325 calories; protein 27.7g; carbohydrates 17g; fat 15.7g; cholesterol 103.3mg; sodium 1565.2mg.

Bacon Stuffed Avocados

Prep:

10 mins

Cook:

20 mins

Total:

30 mins

Servings:

8

Yield:

8 avocado halves

Ingredients

8 slices bacon

2 cloves garlic, chopped

½ cup butter

¼ cup red wine vinegar

1 tablespoon soy sauce

salt to taste

4 avocados - halved, pitted, and peeled

¼ cup brown sugar

Directions

1

Place bacon in a large skillet and cook over medium-high heat, turning occasionally, until evenly browned, about 10 – 12 minutes. Drain bacon slices on paper towels; crumble.

2

Mix butter, brown sugar, vinegar, soy sauce, and garlic in a saucepan; cook and stir mixture over medium heat until sugar is dissolved, about 10 minutes.

3

Sprinkle avocado halves with salt; fill each half with crumbled bacon. Drizzle sauce over filled avocados.

Nutritions

Per Serving: 333 calories; protein 5.7g; carbohydrates 14.1g; fat 30.1g; cholesterol 40.5mg; sodium 413.7mg.

Super Short Ribs

Prep:

30 mins

Cook:

2 hrs

Total:

2 hrs 30 mins

Servings:

8

Yield:

8 servings

Ingredients

1 tablespoon olive oil

2 onions, quartered

1 (8 ounce) can pineapple chunks

1 (14 ounce) can beef broth

½ cup chili sauce

4 ¼ pounds beef short ribs

¼ cup honey

4 cloves garlic, minced

salt and pepper to taste

2 tablespoons chopped fresh parsley, for garnish

3 tablespoons Worcestershire sauce

Directions

1

Preheat oven to 350 degrees F.

2

Heat the oil in a Dutch oven over medium high heat. Add the ribs and brown well on all sides in small batches. Set ribs aside.

3

Add the onions, broth, pineapple, chili sauce, honey, Worcestershire sauce and garlic. Return the ribs to the pot, coating them well with this sauce.

4

Bake, covered, at 350 degrees F for 1 hour. Remove cover, season with salt and pepper to taste, and bake for 1 more hour. Garnish with the parsley.

Nutritions

Per Serving: 600 calories; protein 24.3g; carbohydrates 21.7g; fat 46.1g; cholesterol 99.1mg; sodium 507.7mg.

Salmon Pie

Prep:

20 mins

Cook:

1 hr 25 mins

Total:

1 hr 45 mins

Servings:

6

Yield:

6 to 8 servings

Ingredients

2 (9 inch) unbaked pie crusts

2 onions, thinly sliced

⅔ cup white rice

1 ⅓ cups water

¼ pound fresh mushrooms, sliced

1 tablespoon butter

2 (6 ounce) cans salmon, drained and mashed

⅔ cup shredded Cheddar cheese

1 (10.75 ounce) can condensed cream of mushroom soup

Directions

1

In a medium saucepan cook the rice with the water.

2

Preheat oven to 450 degrees F.

3

Line a pie plate with pastry and set aside.

4

In a large saucepan over medium heat, saute the onions and mushrooms in the butter until soft.

5

Combine the cooked rice with the mushroom soup and spread half of the mixture over the bottom of the pie shell. Spread the mashed salmon over the rice mixture. Top with the sauteed mushroom/onion mixture and then top with the remaining rice mixture. Sprinkle with grated cheese and cover with pastry. Seal edges and pierce top.

6

Bake at 450 degrees F for 11 minutes. Reduce heat to 350 degrees F and continue to bake for another 30 to 35 minutes.

Nutritions

Per Serving: 594 calories; protein 20.9g; carbohydrates 52.6g; fat 33g; cholesterol 53mg; sodium 821.6mg.

Grilled Spicy Shrimp

Prep:

5 mins

Cook:

5 mins

Total:

10 mins

Servings:

4

Yield:

4 servings

Ingredients

1 pound peeled and deveined shrimp

1 teaspoon smoked paprika

½ teaspoon garlic powder

½ teaspoon onion powder

¼ cup Sriracha chile sauce

½ teaspoon ground cumin

½ teaspoon chili powder

Directions

1

Preheat an outdoor grill for medium-high heat and lightly oil the grate.

2

Put shrimp in a large bowl; add chile sauce, paprika, garlic powder, onion powder, chili powder, and cumin and toss to coat.

3

Place shrimp onto the preheated grill using large tongs and cook until they are bright pink on the outside and the meat is no longer transparent in the center, 3 to 4 minutes.

Nutritions

Per Serving: 101 calories; protein 18.8g; carbohydrates 2.6g; fat 1.1g; cholesterol 172.6mg; sodium 837.4mg.

Classic Shrimp Scampi

Prep:

15 mins

Cook:

10 mins

Total:

25 mins

Servings:

4

Yield:

4 servings

Ingredients

1 (8 ounce) package angel hair pasta

¾ cup grated Parmesan cheese

½ cup butter

1 pound shrimp, peeled and deveined

1 cup dry white wine

¼ teaspoon ground black pepper

4 cloves minced garlic

1 tablespoon chopped fresh parsley

Directions

1

Bring a large pot of salted water to a boil. Stir in pasta and return pot to boil. Cook until al dente. Drain well.

2

Melt butter in a large saucepan over medium heat. Stir in garlic and shrimp. Cook, stirring constantly, for 4 to 5 minutes.

3

Stir in wine and pepper. Bring to a boil and cook for 30 seconds while stirring constantly.

4

Mix shrimp with drained pasta in a serving bowl. Sprinkle with cheese and parsley. Serve immediately.

Nutritions

Per Serving: 606 calories; protein 35.3g; carbohydrates 35.5g; fat 30.8g; cholesterol 246.7mg; sodium 680.1mg.

Blackened Tuna

Prep:

10 mins

Cook:

10 mins

Total:

20 mins

Servings:

6

Yield:

6 servings

Ingredients

1 ½ pounds fresh tuna steaks, 1 inch thick

2 tablespoons olive oil

2 tablespoons butter

2 tablespoons Cajun seasoning

Directions

1

Generously coat tuna with Cajun seasoning.

2

Heat oil and butter in a large skillet over high heat. When oil is nearly smoking, place steaks in pan. Cook on one side for 3 to 4 minutes, or until blackened. Turn steaks, and cook for 3 to 5 minutes, or to desired doneness.

Nutritions

Per Serving: 243 calories; protein 26.7g; carbohydrates 1.1g; fat 14g; cholesterol 53.5mg; sodium 545.6mg.

Grilled Red Lobster Tails

Prep:

15 mins

Cook:

12 mins

Total:

27 mins

Servings:

2

Yield:

2 servings

Ingredients

1 tablespoon lemon juice

½ cup olive oil

1 teaspoon paprika

2 (10 ounce) rock lobster tails

⅛ teaspoon white pepper

⅛ teaspoon garlic powder

1 teaspoon salt

Directions

1

Preheat grill for high heat.

2

Squeeze lemon juice into a small bowl, and slowly whisk in olive oil. Whisk in salt, paprika, white pepper, and garlic powder. Split lobster tails lengthwise with a large knife, and brush flesh side of tail with marinade.

3

Lightly oil grill grate. Place tails, flesh side down, on preheated grill. Cook for 10 to 12 minutes, turning once, and basting frequently with marinade. Discard any remaining marinade. Lobster is done when opaque and firm to the touch.

Nutritions

Per Serving: 742 calories; protein 44.3g; carbohydrates 4.3g; fat 60.9g; cholesterol 169.3mg; sodium 2036mg.

Ahi Tuna Steaks

Prep:

5 mins

Cook:

12 mins

Total:

17 mins

Servings:

2

Yield:

2 servings

Ingredients

2 (5 ounce) ahi tuna steaks
¼ teaspoon cayenne pepper
1 teaspoon whole peppercorns
½ tablespoon butter
2 tablespoons olive oil
1 teaspoon kosher salt

Directions

1

Season the tuna steaks with salt and cayenne pepper.

2

Melt the butter with the olive oil in a skillet over medium-high heat. Cook the peppercorns in the mixture until they soften and pop, about 5 minutes. Gently place the seasoned tuna in the skillet and cook to desired doneness, 1 1/2 minutes per side for rare.

Nutritions

Per Serving: 301 calories; protein 33.3g; carbohydrates 0.7g; fat 17.8g; cholesterol 71.4mg; sodium 1033.6mg.

Keto Ceviche

Prep:

30 mins

Cook:

5 mins

Additional:

1 hr

Total:

1 hr 35 mins

Servings:

12

Yield:

12 servings

Ingredients

½ pound sea scallops

½ cup fresh lime juice

1 finely chopped red bell pepper

2 tablespoons fresh orange juice

1 tablespoon grated orange zest

½ cup halved, thinly sliced red onion

1 finely chopped yellow bell pepper

1 cup diced seeded tomato

1 small serrano chile pepper, seeded and minced

½ pound shrimp, peeled and deveined

½ cup coarsely chopped fresh cilantro

kosher salt to taste

1 avocado, diced

1 tablespoon olive oil

⅛ teaspoon ground cumin

Directions

1

Remove the tough side muscles from scallops, if necessary; slice
scallops in half horizontally.

2

Fill a 1-quart saucepan 3/4 full with salted water and bring it to a boil.
Add scallops and reduce heat to a bare simmer. Poach scallops until
just cooked through, about 1 minute. Use a slotted spoon to transfer
the scallops to a bowl of ice water to stop the cooking process.

3

Return the water to a boil and poach shrimp in the same manner,
transferring them to a bowl of ice water after they become opaque
inside and turn pink, 2 to 3 minutes.

4

Drain the scallops and shrimp well and pat dry; place them in a glass
or ceramic bowl and pour in lime juice and orange juice. Cover and
refrigerate for 30 minutes.

5

Pour off most of the juice from the seafood (just leave it moist) and
mix in orange zest, red onion, red and yellow bell peppers, tomato,
chile pepper, cilantro, salt, cumin, and cayenne pepper. Refrigerate an
additional 30 minutes. Just before serving, gently mix in avocado and
drizzle the ceviche with olive oil. Serve in martini glasses or stemmed
margarita glasses.

Nutritions

Per Serving: 83 calories; protein 7.3g; carbohydrates 5.1g; fat 4.1g; cholesterol 36.6mg; sodium 109.4mg.

Taco Fishbowl

Prep:

15 mins

Cook:

17 mins

Total:

32 mins

Servings:

24

Yield:

24 mini taco cups

Ingredients

cooking spray

½ cup salsa

2 cups shredded Mexican cheese blend

2 tablespoons taco seasoning mix

24 wonton wrappers

1 pound ground beef

Directions

1

Preheat the oven to 375 degrees F. Spray a 24-cup mini muffin tin with cooking spray.

2

Heat a large skillet over medium-high heat. Cook and stir beef in the hot skillet until browned and crumbly, 6 to 7 minutes. Drain and discard grease. Mix in salsa and taco seasoning.

3

Line each muffin cup with a wonton wrapper. Add about 1 tablespoon taco beef to each cup. Top with 1 tablespoon shredded Mexican cheese blend.

4

Bake in the preheated oven until wonton wrappers are browned and crispy and cheese is melted, 12 to 15 minutes.

Nutritions

Per Serving: 108 calories; protein 6.4g; carbohydrates 5.8g; fat 6.5g; cholesterol 22.8mg; sodium 226.8mg.

Parchment Baked Salmon

Prep:

15 mins

Cook:

25 mins

Total:

40 mins

Servings:

2

Yield:

2 servings

Ingredients

1 (8 ounce) salmon fillet
1 lemon, thinly sliced
¼ cup chopped basil leaves
olive oil cooking spray
salt and ground black pepper to taste

Directions

1

Place an oven rack in the lowest position in oven and preheat oven to
400 degrees F.

2

Place salmon fillet with skin side down in the middle of a large piece
of parchment paper; season with salt and black pepper. Cut 2 3-inch
slits into the fish with a sharp knife. Stuff chopped basil leaves into the
slits. Spray fillet with cooking spray and arrange lemon slices on top.

3

Fold edges of parchment paper over the fish several times to seal into an airtight packet. Place sealed packet onto a baking sheet.

4

Bake fish on the bottom rack of oven until salmon flakes easily and meat is pink and opaque with an interior of slightly darker pink color, about 25 minutes. An instant-read meat thermometer inserted into the thickest part of the fillet should read at least 145 degrees F. To serve, cut the parchment paper open and remove lemon slices before plating fish.

Nutritions

Per Serving: 175 calories; protein 24.8g; carbohydrates 6.1g; fat 6.9g; cholesterol 49.9mg; sodium 48.3mg

Smoked Salmon and Lettuce Bites

Prep:

20 mins

Total:

20 mins

Servings:

6

Yield:

6 servings

Ingredients

2 cups mayonnaise

1 (3 ounce) package smoked salmon, flaked

½ lemon, juiced

2 tablespoons chopped capers

2 Granny Smith apples, cored and sliced

1 ½ cups sweet corn

3 tablespoons chopped fresh dill

Directions

1

Mix mayonnaise, lemon juice, dill, and capers together in a large bowl until smooth. Add apples, corn, and smoked salmon; toss gently until evenly coated. Chill before serving.

Nutritions

Per Serving: 603 calories; protein 4.9g; carbohydrates 17.8g; fat 59.2g; cholesterol 31.1mg; sodium 615.7mg.

CHAPTER 5: DINNER

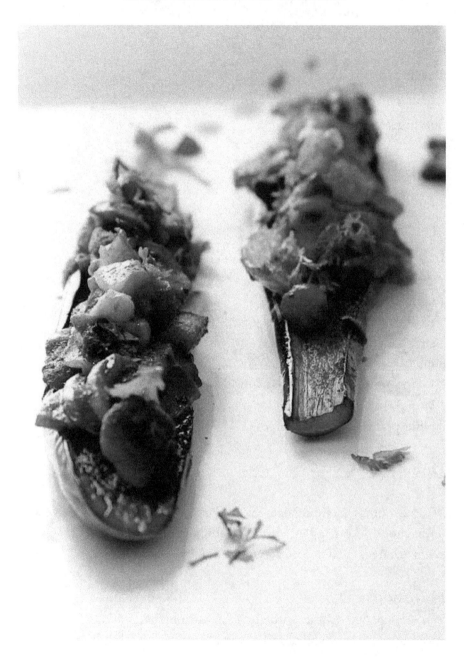

South-American Shrimp

Prep:

10 mins

Cook:

20 mins

Total:

30 mins

Servings:

3

Yield:

3 servings

Ingredients

1 (12 fluid ounce) can evaporated milk
½ cup yellow grits
½ cup chicken broth
1 tablespoon salted butter
⅓ cup grated sharp Cheddar cheese
3 slices bacon
¾ cup frozen bell peppers
⅓ pound frozen medium shrimp - thawed, shelled, and deveined
½ teaspoon taco seasoning mix
2 teaspoons hot sauce, or to taste (Optional)

Directions

1

Combine evaporated milk, grits, chicken broth, and butter in a saucepan over medium-high heat; bring to a boil. Cook, stirring constantly, until thickened, 5 to 7 minutes. Add Cheddar cheese and stir until incorporated. Remove from the heat and set aside.

2

Place bacon in a large skillet and cook over medium-high heat, turning occasionally, until crisp and browned, about 3 minutes per side. Drain bacon slices on paper towels and chop when cool enough to handle.

3

Add bell peppers to the bacon grease. Add shrimp and taco seasoning. Cook and stir until peppers are heated through and shrimp are bright pink on the outside and the meat is opaque, 3 to 5 minutes. Stir in chopped bacon.

4

Place a dollop of grits in each bowl and top with shrimp mixture and hot sauce.

Nutrition

Per Serving: 469 calories; protein 27.2g; carbohydrates 39.7g; fat 22.3g; cholesterol 147.5mg; sodium 866.7mg.

Prosciutto Eggplant Boats

Ingredients

A large eggplant
Prosciutto ham – 6 large slices (cut in half to make 12 rolls)
Ricotta – normal sized tub
Spinach – normal sized bag
Shredded cheese mixture – I used one that had Cheddar, Gouda and
something else (it was in Greek!)
Parmesan – grated
Jar of pasta sauce
Angel hair pasta or thin spaghetti (another side note – Italy doesn't sell
'angel hair' – An American invention perhaps?!)
Olive oil
Seasoning – salt and pepper

Directions

ack on a cookie sheet, take 20 minutes flipping half way at 220 C / 430
F

You want the eggplant to be flimsy enough to roll but not fall apart.
My oven is a boat oven so it takes a lot longer for things to cook…

Lay the eggplant slices on a plate and let them cool

To make the mixture, boil the spinach and drain the water out

In fact, grab the spinach in your hands and squeeze the water out. You
don't want runny water along the bottom of this exquisite dish.

Mix the spinach, ricotta and mixed cheese together. Add some salt and
pepper to taste

In a long baking dish, pour a bit of sauce along the bottom (it helps to ensure the rolls don't stick).

Then, start making your rolls – Start with Eggplant and then…

Add a strip of prosciutto ham and then…

Add a dollop of the cheese/spinach mixture and roll so the seam is at the bottom

Place the roll in the baking dish and then repeat until finished

Then sprinkle some parmesan cheese over the top followed by the rest of the pasta sauce

Sesame Dipping Sauce

Prep:

10 mins

Cook:

5 mins

Total:

15 mins

Servings:

56

Yield:

7 cups

Ingredients

1 tablespoon olive oil
2 tablespoons minced garlic
4 ½ teaspoons red pepper flakes
2 tablespoons minced fresh ginger root
3 cups soy sauce
3 cups honey
1 cup orange juice
1 tablespoon sesame oil
½ lime, juiced
1 tablespoon sesame seeds

Directions

1

Heat the olive oil in a large skillet over medium heat; cook and stir the garlic and red pepper flakes in the hot oil until fragrant, 2 to 3 minutes. Add the ginger, soy sauce, honey, orange juice, sesame oil, lime juice, and sesame seeds; stir. Cook until heated, 2 to 3 minutes more.

Nutrition

Per Serving: 71 calories; protein 1g; carbohydrates 16.8g; fat 0.6g; sodium 774mg.

Pesto Zoodles

Prep:

10 mins

Cook:

10 mins

Total:

20 mins

Servings:

2

Yield:

2 servings

Ingredients

1 tablespoon olive oil
4 small zucchini, cut into noodle-shape strands
½ cup drained and rinsed canned garbanzo beans (chickpeas)
3 tablespoons pesto, or to taste
salt and ground black pepper to taste
2 tablespoons shredded white Cheddar cheese, or to taste

Directions

1

Heat olive oil in a skillet over medium heat; cook and stir zucchini until tender and liquid has evaporated, 5 to 10 minutes.

2

Stir garbanzo beans and pesto into zucchini; lower heat to medium-low. Cook and stir until garbanzo beans are warm and zucchini is evenly coated, about 5 minutes; season with salt and pepper.

3

Transfer zucchini mixture to serving bowls and top with white Cheddar cheese.

Nutrition

Per Serving: 319 calories; protein 12.1g; carbohydrates 23.1g; fat 21.3g; cholesterol 16.2mg; sodium 510.8mg.

Pepperon Fat Head Pizza

INGREDIENTS

For the Crust

1 ¼ cups shredded mozzarella cheese
2 tablespoons cream cheese
1 whole egg
¾ cup almond flour
2 tablespoons parmesan cheese, grated

For the Sauce
2 ounces tomato paste (mixed with water to thin out)
½ tablespoon garlic salt
2 tablespoons fresh basil
1 teaspoon fresh garlic, minced
½ teaspoon dried oregano
For the Toppings
2 tablespoons parmesan cheese
½ cup shredded mozzarella cheese
2 tablespoons Kalamata olives
20 slices uncured pepperoni

Directions

Preheat oven to 425F
Microwave shredded mozzarella cheese and cream cheese for 35
seconds, until melted. Mix in the egg, then almond flour. Knead the
dough till it is well mixed. You may need to microwave it for another
10-20 seconds to be able to blend it thoroughly.
Using your (oiled) hands, spread the dough out onto a parchment
paper lined pizza pan and bake for 8 minutes.

Mix all the sauce ingredients together while the pizza crust is baking. Pull out the pizza dough, add the sauce and your desired toppings. Bake for an additional 6-7 minutes. Allow to cool slightly, cut and serve. Enjoy!

Mushroom Lettuce Wraps

Prep:

40 mins

Cook:

20 mins

Total:

1 hr

Servings:

4

Yield:

4 servings

Ingredients

2 cups water

2 ounces mai fun (angel hair) rice noodles

1 teaspoon vegetable oil

4 shiitake mushrooms, sliced

2 teaspoons vegetable oil

1 (16 ounce) package ground turkey

6 green onions, chopped

¼ cup chopped water chestnuts

4 teaspoons finely minced fresh ginger root

2 teaspoons minced garlic

3 tablespoons soy sauce

2 tablespoons brown sugar

1 tablespoon rice vinegar

1 teaspoon sesame oil

1 teaspoon finely grated orange zest

12 leaves green leaf lettuce

Toppings

½ cup bean sprouts

1 carrot, grated

½ cup salted peanuts

½ cup chopped fresh cilantro

½ cup sweet chili sauce

Directions

1

Bring 2 cups of water to a boil in a small saucepan. Turn off heat; stir in rice noodles. Cover, and allow noodles to soak until soft, 5 to 7 minutes. Rinse with cold water. Drain well.

2

Heat 1 teaspoon of the oil in a large skillet over medium-high heat. Cook the mushrooms in the hot oil until they are browned and softened, about 2 minutes. Remove the mushrooms from the pan. Reserve.

3

Heat the remaining 2 teaspoons of oil in the pan. Cook and stir the turkey in the oil until it is no longer pink, 5 to 7 minutes. Stir in the green onions, water chestnuts, ginger, and garlic; continue to cook for 1 minute. Mix in the reserved mushrooms, soy sauce, and brown sugar. Simmer briefly to combine the flavors. Take the pan off the heat; stir in the rice vinegar, sesame oil, and orange zest.

4

To assemble lettuce wraps, place a bit of turkey filling on each lettuce leaf. Top each with cooked noodles, and a sprinkle of bean sprouts, carrots, peanuts, and cilantro. Serve with sweet chili sauce for dipping.

Nutrition

Per Serving: 481 calories; protein 29.9g; carbohydrates 43.5g; fat 22.4g; cholesterol 83.9mg; sodium 1283.8mg.

Garam Masala

Prep:

15 mins

Cook:

6 mins

Additional:

20 mins

Total:

41 mins

Servings:

12

Yield:

1 /2 cup

Ingredients

¼ cup black cumin seed
2 large bay leaves, crushed
2 tablespoons green cardamom seeds
¼ cup black peppercorns
1 ½ teaspoons whole cloves
1 tablespoon fennel seed
1 teaspoon chopped fresh mace
4 cinnamon sticks, broken
1 pinch ground nutmeg

Directions
1

Heat a small skillet over medium heat; add cumin, bay leaves. cardamom, peppercorns, cloves, fennel seed, mace, and cinnamon sticks and dry roast until fragrant, 6 to 10 minutes.

2

Allow to cool; add nutmeg. Grind the spices into a fine powder using a spice grinder or coffee grinder. Store in an airtight container.

Nutrition

Per Serving: 24 calories; protein 0.8g; carbohydrates 4.1g; fat 0.7g; sodium 5.6mg.

Caprese Quiche

Prep:

15 mins

Cook:

1 hr

Total:

1 hr 15 mins

Servings:

8

Yield:

1 9-inch quiche

Ingredients

1 (9 inch) refrigerated pie crust
2 tablespoons olive oil
¼ cup diced onion
8 large eggs
¼ teaspoon lemon juice
10 leaves chopped fresh basil
¼ teaspoon salt
1 pinch ground black pepper
2 tomatoes, diced
1 (12 ounce) package fresh mozzarella cheese

Directions

1

Preheat oven to 350 degrees F (175 degrees C). Place pie crust on a pie pan or baking dish.

2

Heat olive oil in a skillet over medium heat. Cook and stir onion until softened and translucent, about 5 minutes. Reduce heat to medium-low, and continue cooking and stirring until the onion is very tender and dark brown, 15 to 20 minutes more.

3

Spread mozzarella cheese and tomatoes over the bottom of the pie crust. Whisk eggs, lemon juice, basil, salt, black pepper, and caramelized onion in a large bowl; pour mixture over cheese and tomatoes.

4

Bake in preheated oven until eggs are set and crust is flaky, 30 to 40 minutes.

Nutrition

Per Serving: 331 calories; protein 18.4g; carbohydrates 13.6g; fat 22.7g; cholesterol 213.2mg; sodium 524.7mg.

Kung Pao Tofu Stir-Fry

Prep:

35 mins

Cook:

46 mins

Additional:

45 mins

Total:

2 hrs 6 mins

Servings:

4

Yield:

4 servings

Ingredients

1 (16 ounce) package firm tofu, cut into 3 slices
1 cup low-sodium soy sauce, divided
1 (1 inch) piece ginger, finely grated
1 tablespoon canola oil
1 yellow onion, sliced
1 large green bell pepper, cut into chunks
2 small zucchini, chopped
6 small mushrooms, chopped
3 tablespoons rice wine vinegar
1 tablespoon Asian hot-chile sauce
2 tablespoons crushed roasted peanuts

Directions

1

Lay tofu slices on a paper towel-lined plate and cover with more paper towels. Put a heavy object on top to press out excess water, about 15 minutes; drain and discard the accumulated liquid.

2

Mix 1/2 cup soy sauce and ginger in a large dish. Add tofu slices and let marinate, about 15 minutes.

3

Preheat oven to 350 degrees F (175 degrees C). Line a baking sheet with parchment paper.

4

Flip tofu slices and let marinate on second side, about 15 minutes more. Remove tofu from marinade and place on prepared baking sheet.

5

Bake in the preheated oven until dry, flipping once halfway through, about 40 minutes. Cut into smaller pieces.

6

Heat oil in a wok or large skillet over medium-high heat. Add onion and green bell pepper; cook until onion is slightly translucent, 3 to 5 minutes. Add zucchini and mushrooms; cook and stir until lightly browned, 2 to 3 minutes. Stir in baked tofu.

7

Mix remaining 1/2 cup soy sauce, rice wine vinegar, and chile sauce in a small bowl. Pour into the wok and stir until onion and tofu mixture is well-coated, about 1 minute. Garnish with roasted peanuts.

Nutrition

Per Serving: 213 calories; protein 15.7g; carbohydrates 18.3g; fat 10.6g; sodium 2183.5mg.

Meatless Meatballs

Prep:

15 mins

Cook:

1 hr 20 mins

Total:

1 hr 35 mins

Servings:

20

Yield:

100 small meatballs

Ingredients

4 cups shredded mozzarella cheese
8 eggs
2 cups cracker crumbs
1 ½ cups finely ground pecans
1 (1 ounce) package dry onion soup mix
2 teaspoons celery salt
vegetable oil for frying
1 (10.75 ounce) can condensed cream of mushroom soup
22 fluid ounces milk

Directions

1

Combine mozzarella cheese, eggs, cracker crumbs, pecans, onion soup mix, and celery salt in a large bowl. Form mixture into small meatballs.

2

Heat oil in a deep-fryer or large saucepan. Cook meatballs in batches until browned and crispy, about 5 minutes. Drain on a baking sheet lined paper towels.

3

Transfer meatballs to a large slow cooker. Cover with cream of mushroom soup. Use the empty can to measure and pour in milk. Cook on Low until flavors combine and soup mixture thickens, 30 minutes to 2 hours.

Nutrition

Per Serving: 246 calories; protein 11.1g; carbohydrates 14.4g; fat 16.3g; cholesterol 91.5mg; sodium 555.3mg.

Zoodle Bolognese

Prep:

20 mins

Cook:

2 hrs 40 mins

Total:

3 hrs

Servings:

8

Yield:

8 servings

Ingredients

4 ounces pancetta bacon, finely diced

3 carrots, finely diced

3 stalks celery, finely diced

2 onions, finely diced

3 tablespoons extra-virgin olive oil

1 pound 85% lean ground beef

1 pound ground pork

½ cup dry white wine

1 (28 ounce) can San Marzano whole peeled tomatoes, drained

½ teaspoon ground nutmeg

½ teaspoon salt

¼ teaspoon crushed red pepper

1 cup beef stock

¼ cup heavy cream

1 (16 ounce) box tagliatelle pasta

¼ cup grated Parmesan cheese, or to taste

Directions

1

Cook pancetta in a pan over medium heat until it has released its fat and is crisp, 7 to 8 minutes. Add carrots, celery, and onions and cook until the vegetables soften and the onions are translucent, 7 to 8 minutes. Set aside.

2

Heat olive oil in a 4-quart pot over medium heat. Break ground beef and pork into small chunks and add them to the pot; cook, stirring lightly, until browned, 7 to 8 minutes.

3

Stir the pancetta-vegetable mixture into the ground meat. Add wine. Reduce heat to medium-low and stir, breaking up the meat until finely ground, wine has evaporated, and the pot is almost dry, 13 to 15 minutes. Add tomatoes, nutmeg, salt, and red pepper. Use the back of a spoon to break up the tomatoes and continue to break down the meat mixture into very small bits, about 5 minutes.

4

Pour beef stock and heavy cream into the pot and reduce heat to the lowest setting. Leave to simmer, partially covered, stirring occasionally, for at least 2 hours.

5

Meanwhile, fill a large pot with lightly salted water and bring to a rolling boil. Cook tagliatelle at a boil until tender yet firm to the bite, about 8 minutes. Reserve 1 cup of pasta water and drain well.

6

Stir pasta into the Bolognese sauce and mix well, adding a little reserved pasta water if needed to develop a satiny coating. Top with grated Parmesan cheese.

Nutrition

Per Serving: 607 calories; protein 34.3g; carbohydrates 54.9g; fat 26.9g; cholesterol 94.6mg; sodium 543.9mg.

Harissa Chicken

Prep:

20 mins

Cook:

10 mins

Additional:

4 hrs

Total:

4 hrs 30 mins

Servings:

4

Yield:

4 servings

Ingredients

2 tablespoons smoked paprika
2 cloves garlic, minced
1 teaspoon ground cumin
1 teaspoon caraway seeds
1 chipotle pepper in adobo sauce
1 teaspoon adobo sauce from chipotle peppers
4 skinless, boneless chicken breast halves
1 tablespoon extra-virgin olive oil
salt and black pepper to taste

Directions

1

Place the smoked paprika, garlic, cumin, caraway seeds, chipotle pepper, and adobo sauce into a mortar, and grind together with a pestle to make a paste. Smear the paste all over the chicken breasts, place into a bowl, cover, and refrigerate at least 4 hours or overnight.

2

Preheat an outdoor grill for medium heat, and lightly oil the grate.

3

Remove chicken from marinade, and discard the excess marinade. Brush the chicken breasts with olive oil, and sprinkle with salt and pepper. Grill the chicken breasts until the meat shows grill marks and the inside is no longer pink, about 5 minutes per side.

Nutrition

Per Serving: 178 calories; protein 28g; carbohydrates 3.2g; fat 5.6g; cholesterol 68.4mg; sodium 100.8mg.

Seitan and Cauliflower

Prep:

20 mins

Cook:

20 mins

Total:

40 mins

Servings:

2

Yield:

2 servings

Ingredients

1 tablespoon vegetable oil

1 (8 ounce) package seitan, sliced

1 ½ teaspoons vegetable oil

½ cup mushrooms, cut into bite-size pieces, or to taste

¼ cup all-purpose flour

1 cup water, or as needed

2 cubes vegetable bouillon

1 pinch cayenne pepper, or to taste (Optional)

1 pinch dried rosemary, or to taste (Optional)

1 pinch dried thyme, or to taste (Optional)

1 small head cauliflower, cut into bite-size pieces

Directions

1

Heat 1 tablespoon oil in a skillet over medium-high heat; saute seitan until cooked through and browned, about 5 minutes. Remove skillet from heat and cover with a lid.

2

Heat 1 1/2 teaspoons vegetable oil in a small saucepan over medium-high heat; saute mushrooms until lightly browned, about 3 minutes. Whisk flour into mushroom mixture using a fork until mushrooms are coated, 2 to 3 minutes.

3

Slowly pour water into mushroom-flour mixture while constantly stirring with a fork until smooth; add bouillon cubes. Decrease heat to medium-low and continue stirring until bouillon is dissolved and gravy is smooth, 5 to 10 minutes more. Season gravy with cayenne pepper, rosemary, and thyme.

4

Mix cauliflower into seitan; cook and stir over medium heat until cauliflower is slightly softened, 3 to 5 minutes. Add gravy; bring to a boil, reduce heat, cover skillet, and simmer, stirring occasionally, until seitan is softened, 7 to 10 minutes.

Nutrition

Per Serving: 347 calories; protein 30.8g; carbohydrates 30.4g; fat 12.7g; sodium 371.2mg.

Mushroom Risotto

Prep:

10 mins

Cook:

35 mins

Total:

45 mins

Servings:

4

Yield:

4 servings

Ingredients

1 tablespoon olive oil
3 small onions, finely chopped
1 clove garlic, crushed
1 teaspoon minced fresh parsley
1 teaspoon minced celery
salt and pepper to taste
1 ½ cups sliced fresh mushrooms
1 cup whole milk
¼ cup heavy cream
1 cup rice
5 cups vegetable stock
1 teaspoon butter
1 cup grated Parmesan cheese

Directions

1

Heat olive oil in a large skillet over medium-high heat. Saute the onion and garlic in the olive oil until onion is tender and garlic is lightly browned. Remove garlic, and stir in the parsley, celery, salt, and pepper. Cook until celery is tender, then add the mushrooms. Reduce heat to low, and continue cooking until the mushrooms are soft.

2

Pour the milk and cream into the skillet, and stir in the rice. Heat to a simmer. Stir the vegetable stock into the rice one cup at a time, until it is absorbed.

3

When the rice has finished cooking, stir in the butter and Parmesan cheese, and remove from heat. Serve hot.

Nutrition

Per Serving: 439 calories; protein 16.9g; carbohydrates 48.7g; fat 19.5g; cholesterol 49.9mg; sodium 767.6mg.

Chicken Cordon Blue Casserole

Prep:

15 mins

Cook:

40 mins

Total:

55 mins

Servings:

8

Yield:

8 servings

Ingredients

1 egg

½ cup milk

2 pounds skinless, boneless chicken breast halves - cut into chunks

1 cup plain dried bread crumbs

1 cup oil for frying

8 ounces Swiss cheese, cubed

8 ounces cubed ham

1 (10.75 ounce) can condensed cream of chicken soup

1 cup milk

Directions

1

Preheat oven to 350 degrees F (175 degrees C).

2

Beat egg and 1/2 cup milk together until combined. Stir in the chicken chunks to coat, then drain, and coat with bread crumbs. Heat oil in a large skillet to 375 degrees F (190 degrees C). Fry breaded chicken cubes in hot oil until golden brown on all sides, then remove, and drain on paper towels.

3

Place chicken cubes in a glass baking dish, along with the Swiss cheese, and ham. Stir together the soup with 1 cup milk, pour over casserole.

4

Bake in preheated oven until golden brown and bubbly, about 30 minutes.

Nutrition

Per Serving: 500 calories; protein 36.2g; carbohydrates 24.2g; fat 28g; cholesterol 137.4mg; sodium 1016.5mg.

Arugula and Hummus Mini Pizzas

Prep:

10 mins

Total:

10 mins

Servings:

1

Yield:

1 pizza

Ingredients

2 tablespoons hummus, or to taste

1 naan bread

1 cup arugula, or to taste

1 date, pitted and finely chopped

2 teaspoons pumpkin seeds

1 teaspoon balsamic vinegar, or to taste

Directions

1

Spread hummus onto naan bread; top with arugula, date, and pumpkin seeds. Drizzle balsamic vinegar over pizza.

Nutrition

Per Serving: 350 calories; protein 14.4g; carbohydrates 56.8g; fat 8.5g; cholesterol 10mg; sodium 424mg.

Punjabi Chicken in Thick Gravy

Prep:

25 mins

Cook:

1 hr 5 mins

Total:

1 hr 30 mins

Servings:

8

Yield:

8 servings

Ingredients

2 tablespoons vegetable oil
2 tablespoons ghee (clarified butter)
8 chicken legs, skin removed
1 teaspoon cumin seeds
1 onion, finely chopped
5 cloves garlic, minced
2 tablespoons minced fresh ginger root
1 small tomato, coarsely chopped
1 tablespoon tomato paste
1 tablespoon garam masala
1 tablespoon ground turmeric
1 teaspoon salt, or to taste
1 serrano chile pepper, seeded and minced
1 cup water
¼ cup chopped fresh cilantro

Directions

1

Heat the oil and ghee in a large pot over medium heat. Cook the cumin seeds in the oil until the seeds begin to change color.

2

Stir in chopped onion onion; cook and stir until onion has softened and turned translucent, about 5 minutes. Add the garlic and ginger; continue cooking until the onions brown, about 5 minutes more.

3

Mix in the chopped tomato, tomato paste, garam masala, turmeric, salt, serrano pepper, and water; simmer 5 minutes. Lay the chicken into the sauce; mix gently to coat the legs. Cover pan and reduce heat to medium-low. Cook until chicken is no longer pink near the bone, about 40 minutes. Garnish with cilantro to serve.

Nutrition

Per Serving: 325 calories; protein 27.7g; carbohydrates 4.3g; fat 21.5g; cholesterol 102.2mg; sodium 394.5mg.

Chargrilled Chili Chicken

Servings:

5

Yield:

4 servings

Ingredients

3 tablespoons vegetable oil
2 cloves garlic, minced
1 green bell pepper, chopped
1 onion, chopped
1 stalk celery, sliced
¼ pound mushrooms, chopped
1 pound skinless, boneless chicken breast halves - cut into bite size pieces
1 tablespoon chili powder
1 teaspoon dried oregano
1 teaspoon ground cumin
½ teaspoon paprika
½ teaspoon cocoa powder
¼ teaspoon salt
1 pinch crushed red pepper flakes
1 pinch ground black pepper
1 (14.5 ounce) can whole peeled tomatoes with juice
1 (19 ounce) can kidney beans, drained and rinsed

Directions

1

In a large skillet heat 2 tablespoons of the oil over medium heat. Saute the garlic, bell pepper, onion, celery and mushrooms for 5 minutes. Set aside.

2

Add the remaining 1 tablespoon of oil to the skillet and brown the chicken over high heat until it is golden brown and firm on the outside. Return the vegetable mixture to the skillet.

3

Add the chili powder, cumin, oregano, paprika, cocoa powder, salt, hot pepper flakes and ground black pepper to the skillet. Stir for a few minutes to prevent burning. Add the tomatoes and beans, bring all to a boil and reduce heat to low. Cover the skillet and simmer for 15 minutes, then remove cover and simmer for 15 more minutes.

Nutrition

Per Serving: 308 calories; protein 29g; carbohydrates 25.9g; fat 10.5g; cholesterol 52.7mg; sodium 547mg.

Baked Cajun Chicken Drumsticks

Prep:

10 mins

Cook:

30 mins

Total:

40 mins

Servings:

8

Yield:

8 drumsticks

Ingredients

8 chicken drumsticks
2 tablespoons vegetable oil
1 teaspoon paprika
½ teaspoon salt
½ teaspoon ground black pepper
½ teaspoon onion powder
½ teaspoon garlic powder
½ teaspoon oregano
½ teaspoon basil
¼ teaspoon ground thyme
¼ teaspoon cayenne pepper

Directions

1

Preheat the oven to 400 degrees F (200 degrees C). Line a baking sheet with aluminum foil.

2

Place chicken in a gallon-sized resealable plastic bag. Drizzle vegetable oil over the chicken. Seal the bag and massage the oil into the chicken.

3

Combine paprika, salt, pepper, onion powder, garlic powder, oregano, basil, thyme, and cayenne pepper in a small bowl. Mix until evenly combined. Pour spice mixture into the bag with the chicken. Seal the bag and toss to coat.

4

Transfer drumsticks to the prepared baking sheet, discarding the plastic bag.

5

Bake until chicken is no longer pink at the bone and the juices run clear, about 25 minutes. An instant-read thermometer inserted near the bone should read 165 degrees F (74 degrees C).

6

For extra crispy skin, set an oven rack about 6 inches from the heat source and preheat the oven's broiler. Broil chicken for 5 minutes.

Nutrition

Per Serving: 170 calories; protein 20.2g; carbohydrates 0.6g; fat 9.2g; cholesterol 66mg; sodium 213.1mg.

Provolone Chicken Bake

Prep:

15 mins

Cook:

30 mins

Total:

45 mins

Servings:

8

Yield:

8 servings

Ingredients

8 skinless, boneless chicken breast halves

1 (16 ounce) package herb seasoned stuffing mix

2 (10.75 ounce) cans condensed cream of chicken soup

10 ¾ fluid ounces white wine

¼ cup melted butter

4 slices provolone cheese, halved

Directions

1

Preheat oven to 350 degrees F.

2

Arrange chicken breast halves in a single layer in a 9x13 inch baking dish. Top each breast half with a half slice of Provolone cheese.

3

In a medium bowl, blend cream of chicken soup and white wine. Pour over the chicken.

4

In a separate medium bowl, mix the butter and stuffing mix. Top the chicken with the stuffing mixture.

5

Bake 30 minutes in the preheated oven, or until chicken is no longer pink and juices run clear.

Nutrition

Per Serving: 555 calories; protein 39.3g; carbohydrates 49.8g; fat 17.3g; cholesterol 99.6mg; sodium 1524.7mg.

Fennel Cucumber Salsa

Prep:

20 mins

Additional:

20 mins

Total:

40 mins

Servings:

16

Yield:

4 cups

Ingredients

1 English cucumber, diced

2 tablespoons honey

1 large fennel bulb, diced

½ red onion, chopped

½ cup pickled banana peppers, diced

salt and pepper to tastE

1 bunch cilantro, chopped

1 avocado - peeled, pitted, and diced

3 tablespoons fresh lemon juice

Directions

1

Combine the cucumber, fennel, avocado, red onion, banana peppers, cilantro, honey, lemon juice, salt, and pepper in a bowl. Allow mixture to sit 20 minutes before serving.

Nutrition

Per Serving: 43 calories; protein 0.9g; carbohydrates 6.8g; fat 2g; sodium 18.4mg.

Peanut Butter French Toast

Prep:

10 mins

Cook:

10 mins

Total:

20 mins

Servings:

2

Yield:

2 servings

Ingredients

½ cup milk

1 tablespoon vegetable oil

3 eggs

¼ cup peanut butter

¼ teaspoon ground cinnamon

4 slices bread

2 tablespoons white sugar

Directions

1

Whisk together milk, eggs, peanut butter, sugar, vanilla extract, and cinnamon in a large bowl.

2

Heat the oil in a griddle or frying pan over medium heat.

3

Dunk each slice of bread in egg mixture, soaking both sides. Place in pan, and cook on both sides until golden, about 3 to 5 minutes per side. Serve hot.

Nutrition

Per Serving: 573 calories; protein 23.4g; carbohydrates 47.9g; fat 33.4g; cholesterol 283.9mg; sodium 618.7mg.

Baked Maple Glazed Ribs

Prep:

20 mins

Cook:

2 hrs

Total:

2 hrs 20 mins

Servings:

6

Yield:

6 servings

Ingredients

3 pounds pork spareribs, cut into serving size pieces

1 cup pure maple syrup

3 tablespoons ketchup

2 tablespoons soy sauce

1 tablespoon Dijon mustard

1 clove garlic, minced

1 tablespoon Worcestershire sauce

1 teaspoon curry powder

2 green onions, minced

1 tablespoon toasted sesame seeds

3 tablespoons frozen orange juice concentrate

Directions

1

Preheat oven to 350 degrees F. Place ribs meat side up on a rack in a 9x13 inch roasting pan. Cover pan tightly with foil. Bake for 1 1/4 hours.

2

In a saucepan over medium heat, combine maple syrup, orange juice concentrate, ketchup, soy sauce, mustard and Worcestershire sauce. Stir in curry powder, garlic and green onions. Simmer for 15-16 minutes, stirring occasionally.

3

Remove ribs from roasting pan, remove rack, and drain excess fat and drippings. Return ribs to pan, cover with sauce, and bake uncovered for 35 minutes, basting occasionally. Sprinkle with sesame seeds just before serving.

Nutrition

Per Serving: 806 calories; protein 36.2g; carbohydrates 43.1g; fat 54g; cholesterol 181.4mg; sodium 664.4mg.

Skinny Spaghetti Squash Alfredo

Prep:

10 mins

Cook:

1 hr 5 mins

Total:

1 hr 15 mins

Servings:

2

Yield:

2 servings

Ingredients

1 medium spaghetti squash, halved and seeded

1 tablespoon butter

¼ teaspoon kosher salt

3 cloves garlic, minced

1 ½ cups fat-free milk

1 tablespoon cream cheese

1 cup grated Parmesan cheese, or more to taste

2 tablespoons grated Parmesan cheese

2 tablespoons all-purpose flour

⅛ teaspoon ground black pepper

Directions

1

Preheat the oven to 350 degrees F.

2

Place squash, cut-sides down, on a rimmed baking sheet and add water to surround squash.

3

Bake in the preheated oven until tender, about 60 minutes.

4

Gently scrape squash strands into the center of each half using a fork.

5

Melt butter in a small saucepan over medium-low heat. Add garlic to hot butter and cook 1 to 2 minutes. Whisk in flour and cook for another minute while stirring until no lumps remain, 1 to 2 minutes more. Whisk in milk heated through. Add cream cheese and stir until smooth. Stir in Parmesan cheese, salt, and pepper.

6

Spoon hot sauce equally on to each squash half. Gently pull up the squash strands to coat as much as possible with sauce. Top with extra Parmesan cheese if desired.

7

Set an oven rack about 6 inches from the heat source and preheat the oven's broiler. Place squash halves under the broiler until golden and bubbly, 2 to 4 minutes.

Nutrition

Per Serving: 477 calories; protein 27.5g; carbohydrates 42.9g; fat 23.4g; cholesterol 66.5mg; sodium 1128.1mg.

Salisbury Steak

Prep:

15 mins

Cook:

50 mins

Total:

1 hr 5 mins

Servings:

5

Yield:

5 servings

Ingredients

Patties:

1 pound ground sirloin

½ (1 ounce) package dry onion soup mix

½ cup panko bread crumbs

1 egg, beaten

2 tablespoons milk

1 teaspoon Worcestershire sauce

¼ teaspoon ground black pepper

Gravy:

3 tablespoons butter

1 sweet onion, sliced

3 tablespoons all-purpose flour

½ (1 ounce) package dry onion soup mix

2 cups fresh mushrooms, sliced

1 ½ cups beef stock

1 cup water

salt and ground black pepper to taste

Directions

1

Mix ground sirloin, panko bread crumbs, egg, milk, and 1/2 packet onion soup mix, Worcestershire sauce, and black pepper together in a large bowl; shape into 5 patties.

2

Heat a skillet over medium heat. Cook patties in hot skillet until browned, 3 to 4 minutes per side.

3

Melt butter in a separate skillet over medium-high heat. Saute mushrooms and onion in melted butter until tender, 5 to 7 minutes. Stir flour and remaining dry onion soup mix into the mushroom mixture; cook and stir until flour is integrated fully, about 1 minute. Stream beef stock and water over the mushroom mixture while stirring continually; bring to a simmer, reduce heat to medium, and cook, stirring frequently, until the liquid thickens, about 6 minutes. Season with salt and pepper.

4

Lie the browned steaks into the gravy; simmer until steaks are firm and gray in the center, about 30 minutes. An instant-read thermometer inserted into the center should read 160 degrees F.

Nutrition

Per Serving: 367 calories; protein 28.5g; carbohydrates 21.1g; fat 20g; cholesterol 113.5mg; sodium 6585.2mg.

Steak Camitas

Prep:

20 mins

Cook:

1 hr 45 mins

Total:

2 hrs 5 mins

Servings:

6

Yield:

6 servings

Ingredients

2 pounds boneless pork shoulder, cut into 1-inch cubes

Goya Adobo with Pepper

½ medium onion

1 teaspoon Goya Minced Garlic

Water to cover

3 tablespoons Goya Corn Oil

1 ½ cups orange juice

1 (12 ounce) tub Goya Frozen Guacamole, thawed

1 packet Sazon Goya without Annatto

Goya Flour Tortillas, warmed

1 packet Goya Powdered Chicken Bouillon

1 (17.6 ounce) container Goya Salsa Pico de Gallo (Mild)

Directions

1

Season meat with Adobo.

2

In a deep-sided frying pan or casserole, combine pork, onion, garlic, Jalapeno, bouillon. Add water to cover. Bring to boil, cover and simmer on low heat until meat is tender, about 1 hour.

3

Preheat oven to 400 degrees F.

4

Drain pork in colander, discarding vegetables and water.

5

Heat oil in same pan on medium high. Add drained meat and brown, turning occasionally. When meat is browned, add orange juice and Sazon and bring to boil. Place in oven, uncovered, until juice reduces and glazes meat, about 30 minutes. Stir every 5-10 minutes so it doesn't stick and juice evenly coats meat.

6

Serve with Tortillas, Salsa Pico de Gallo and Guacamole.

Honey-Mustard Salmon Fillet with White Wine Sauce

Prep:

15 mins

Cook:

10 mins

Total:

25 mins

Servings:

6

Yield:

2 pounds of salmon

Ingredients

2 pounds salmon fillets

1 tablespoon garlic powder

1 teaspoon kosher salt

1 teaspoon freshly cracked black pepper

4 tablespoons butter, divided

2 tablespoons vegetable oil

2 tablespoons Worcestershire sauce

3 cloves garlic, minced

1 tablespoon balsamic vinegar

4 tablespoons honey mustard

1 tablespoon dried parsley

1 lemon, sliced

2 cups white wine

1 teaspoon cornstarch

1 teaspoon liquid smoke flavoring

Directions

1

Set an oven rack about 6 inches from the heat source and preheat the oven's broiler.

2

Place salmon fillets in an oven-safe dish. Sprinkle with salt and pepper.

3

Melt 2 tablespoons butter in a microwave-safe bowl. Whisk in honey mustard, vegetable oil, Worcestershire sauce, minced garlic, balsamic vinegar, parsley, garlic powder, and liquid smoke. Spoon enough sauce onto the salmon to cover it well; brush sauce around with a basting brush. Top fish with 1/2 the lemon slices.

4

Broil in the preheated oven until fish flakes easily with a fork, about 10 minutes.

5

Melt remaining butter in a small saucepan. Add the remaining salmon glaze and whisk to combine. Add white wine; whisk and reduce by 1/4. Stir in cornstarch; stir until no lumps remain and sauce begins to thicken.

6

Plate the salmon and drizzle the white wine sauce on top.

Nutrition

Per Serving: 468 calories; protein 27.3g; carbohydrates 12.5g; fat 28.4g; cholesterol 95mg; sodium 591mg.

Saucy Salmon with Tarragon

Prep:

20 mins

Cook:

10 mins

Total:

30 mins

Servings:

4

Yield:

4 servings

Ingredients

4 (4 ounce) fillets salmon
salt and ground black pepper to taste
½ cup mayonnaise
2 tablespoons Dijon mustard
2 tablespoons olive oil
4 cloves garlic, minced
2 tablespoons olive oi
1 tablespoon lemon juice
2 tablespoons chopped fresh tarragon
¼ teaspoon salt
¼ teaspoon ground black pepper
1 tablespoon finely grated lemon zest

Directions

1

Prepare a grill for high heat.

2

Season the salmon fillets with salt and pepper and drizzle with olive oil.

3

Whisk together the mayonnaise, mustard, olive oil, garlic, lemon juice, tarragon, salt and pepper; set aside.

4

Lightly oil the grill grate. Cook the salmon on the grill until the fish flakes easily with a fork, 5 to 10 minutes. Place on a serving plate and top with the prepared sauce.

Nutrition

Per Serving: 512 calories; protein 19.9g; carbohydrates 4.3g; fat 46.2g; cholesterol 65.4mg; sodium 543.5mg.

Speedy Tilapia Tacos

Prep:

30 mins

Cook:

25 mins

Total:

55 mins

Servings:

4

Yield:

4 servings

Ingredients

cooking spray

¼ teaspoon fajita seasoning

4 (4 ounce) tilapia fillets

⅛ teaspoon fajita seasoning

2 pineapple rings, cut into chunks

½ small red onion, chopped

1 tablespoon olive oil, divided

12 (6 inch) corn tortillas

¾ cup frozen white corn

¾ cup canned black beans

¼ cup chopped fresh cilantro

1 avocado, sliced

¼ cup sour cream

½ lime, cut into wedges

⅛ head cabbage, chopped

Directions

1

Preheat oven to 350 degrees F. Spray a baking sheet with cooking spray.

2

Sprinkle 1/4 teaspoon fajita seasoning over tilapia fillets and arrange on the prepared baking sheet.

3

Bake tilapia in the preheated oven until fish flakes easily with a fork, 15 to 20 minutes. Remove fish from oven and cut each fillet into 3 pieces.

4

Spray a skillet with cooking spray and add corn, black beans, and 1/8 teaspoon fajita seasoning; cook and stir over medium-high heat until heated through, about 3 minutes. Remove skillet from heat.

5

Spray a separate skillet with cooking spray and add pineapple; cook and stir over medium-high heat until lightly browned, about 2 minutes. Add onion to pineapple; cook and stir until heated through, about 1 minute more. Remove skillet from heat.

6

Pour 1 teaspoon olive oil in a large skillet over high heat; add 4 tortillas and cook until heated through, about 30 seconds per side. Remove tortillas from skillet and repeat cooking the remaining tortillas in the remaining oil.

7

Place a piece of tilapia onto each tortilla and top with corn mixture, pineapple mixture, cilantro, avocado, cabbage, sour cream and a squeeze of lime.

Nutrition

Per Serving: 526 calories; protein 33.2g; carbohydrates 62.3g; fat 18g; cholesterol 47.3mg; sodium 293.4mg.

Prawn Saganaki

Prep:

15 mins

Cook:

35 mins

Total:

50 mins

Servings:

4

Yield:

4 servings

Ingredients

1 tablespoon olive oil

3 cloves garlic, thinly sliced

2 tablespoons tomato paste

1 ½ pounds prawns, peeled and deveined, tail on

½ cup white wine

1 (13.5 ounce) jar tomato and olive pasta sauce (such as Papayiannides® Tomato & Olive & Ouzo Sauce)

½ cup crumbled Greek feta cheese

2 tablespoons chopped fresh flat-leaf parsley

1 red onion, halved and thinly sliced

Directions

1

Preheat oven to 400 degrees F.

2

Heat olive oil in a large skillet over medium heat; cook and stir onion until soft, about 5 minutes. Stir in garlic and cook until fragrant, about 1 minute. Stir tomato paste into onion mixture; cook and stir for 1 minute.

3

Pour wine into tomato mixture; simmer until liquid is reduced by about half, about 5 minutes. Stir tomato sauce into wine mixture and simmer until mixture is thick, about 10 minutes.

4

Spread tomato mixture into the base of a 6-cup baking dish; top with prawns and sprinkle evenly with feta cheese.

5

Bake in the preheated oven until prawns are bright pink on the outside and the meat is no longer transparent in the center, about 10 minutes; top with parsley.

Nutrition

Per Serving: 341 calories; protein 33g; carbohydrates 19.7g; fat 11.5g; cholesterol 277.5mg; sodium 967.5mg.

Wine Shrimp Scampi Pizza

Prep:

20 mins

Cook:

25 mins

Total:

45 mins

Servings:

3

Yield:

3 servings

Ingredients

12 ounces angel hair pasta

½ teaspoon cayenne pepper

¼ cup olive oil

2 tablespoons butter

½ yellow onion, diced

4 cloves garlic, minced

2 tablespoons chopped fresh cilantro

1 small tomato, diced

¼ cup olives, chopped

¼ cup chopped leeks

½ lemon, juiced

2 teaspoons capers

2 teaspoons salt

¼ cup Chardonnay wine

1 pound uncooked medium shrimp, peeled and deveined

¼ cup heavy whipping cream

Directions

1

Bring a large pot of lightly salted water to a boil. Cook angel hair pasta in the boiling water, stirring occasionally, until tender yet firm to the bite, 4 to 5 minutes. Drain.

2

Heat olive oil and butter in a large skillet over medium heat. Add onion and garlic; cook until onion is transparent, about 4 minutes. Add tomato, olives, Chardonnay wine, leeks, lemon juice, capers, salt, and cayenne pepper. Bring to a boil. Mix in shrimp and simmer until pink, about 10 minutes. Stir in heavy whipping cream and cilantro. Serve on top of angel hair pasta.

Nutrition

Per Serving: 796 calories; protein 38.5g; carbohydrates 72.5g; fat 38.8g; cholesterol 277.6mg; sodium 2272.1mg.

Vegetarian Nori Rolls

Prep:

30 mins

Cook:

30 mins

Additional:

1 hr

Total:

2 hrs

Servings:

5

Yield:

5 servings

Ingredients

2 cups uncooked short-grain white rice

2 ¼ cups water

3 ounces firm tofu, cut into 1/2 inch strips

¼ cup soy sauce

2 teaspoons honey

1 teaspoon minced garlic

2 tablespoons rice vinegar

½ avocado, julienned

4 sheets nori seaweed sheets

½ cucumber, julienned

1 small carrot, julienned

Directions

1

In a large saucepan cover rice with water and let stand for 30 minutes.

2

In a shallow dish combine soy sauce, honey and garlic. In this mixture marinate tofu for at least 30 minutes.

3

Bring water and rice to a boil and then reduce heat; simmer for about 20 minutes, or until thick and sticky. In a large glass bowl combine cooked rice with rice vinegar.

4

Place a sheet of nori on a bamboo mat. Working with wet hands, spread 1/4 of the rice evenly over the nori; leave about 1/2 inch on the top edge of the nori. Place 2 strips of marinated tofu end to end about 1 inch from the bottom. Place 2 strips of cucumber next to the tofu, then avocado and carrot.

5

Roll nori tightly from the bottom, using the mat to help make a tight roll. Seal by moistening with water the 1/2 inch at the top. Repeat with remaining ingredients. Slice with a serrated knife into 1 inch thick slices.

Nutrition

Per Serving: 289 calories; protein 8.1g; carbohydrates 53.6g; fat 4.8g; sodium 734.2mg.

Creamy Shrimp Shirataki Noodles

Prep:

15 mins

Cook:

5 mins

Total:

20 mins

Servings:

2

Yield:

2 servings

Ingredients

1 (3 ounce) package ramen noodles (flavor packet discarded)

2 tablespoons chopped dry-roasted peanuts

8 ounces frozen cooked shrimp, thawed

½ cup shredded carrot

½ cup thinly bias-sliced celery

⅓ cup bottled chile-lime vinaigrette

½ cup julienned red bell pepper

2 sprigs fresh mint

Directions

1

Cook ramen according to package directions. Drain in a colander under cold running water until cool; drain again.

2

Toss together ramen, shrimp, bell pepper, carrot, celery, and vinaigrette in a bowl. Top servings with peanuts, mint, and black pepper. Serve cold.

Nutrition

Per Serving: 299 calories; protein 26.9g; carbohydrates 16.6g; fat 13.9g; cholesterol 218.4mg; sodium 866.4mg.

Mahi Mahi Ceviche

Prep:

30 mins

Additional:

1 hr

Total:

1 hr 30 mins

Servings:

6

Yield:

6 servings

Ingredients

¾ pound mahi mahi fillets, diced, or more to taste

⅓ cup lime juice

⅓ cup lemon juice

½ teaspoon salt

1 pinch dried oregano

1 pinch cayenne pepper

½ cup diced avocados

½ cup peeled and seeded diced cucumber

1 tablespoon minced jalapeno pepper

½ cup diced orange segments

½ cup chopped fresh chives

1 tablespoon chopped cilantro

1 tablespoon olive oil

2 tablespoons radishes, sliced

Directions

1

Stir mahi mahi, lime juice, lemon juice, jalapeno pepper, salt, oregano, and cayenne pepper together in a bowl. Press down fish to completely immerse in liquid. Cover the bowl with plastic wrap and press plastic wrap down so that it is touching the fish. Refrigerate for at least 1 hour, or up to 6 hours.

2

Stir avocado, cucumber, orange, chives, radish, cilantro, and olive oil into mahi mahi mixture until completely coated. Season with salt.

Nutrition

Per Serving: 117 calories; protein 11.4g; carbohydrates 6.5g; fat 5.6g; cholesterol 41.5mg; sodium 247mg.

Sea Bass Veracruz

Prep:
30 mins
Cook:
15 mins
Total:
45 mins
Servings:
4
Yield:
4 fillets

Ingredients

2 cups Roma tomatoes, seeded and diced
½ cup chopped pimento-stuffed olives
½ cup cilantro
3 tablespoons lime juice
2 tablespoons capers
6 tablespoons extra-virgin olive oil
¼ cup all-purpose flour
4 (6 ounce) fillets sea bass
salt to taste
ground black pepper to taste
¼ cup chicken broth
2 cups sliced onion
1 tablespoon minced garlic
¼ cup jalapeno pepper, seeded and diced
2 bay leaves
1 teaspoon dried thyme

Directions

1

Preheat the oven to 375 degrees F.

2

Combine tomatoes, olives, cilantro, jalapeno, lime juice, and capers together in a bowl. Place flour in a shallow bowl.

3

Place fish on a flat work surface and season with salt and pepper. Dredge one side of each fillet in flour.

4

Heat oil in a large, ovenproof skillet over medium-high heat. Add fish, flour-side down, and saute for 4 minutes. Transfer to a plate. Stir broth into skillet and scrape the bottom to deglaze. Add 1/2 the tomato mixture. Add onion, garlic, bay leaves, and thyme. Saute 3 minutes more. Nestle fillets into the skillet.

5

Place skillet in the preheated oven and roast until fish flakes easily with a fork, 6 to 7 minutes.

6

Remove and discard bay leaves. Add remaining tomato mixture to the skillet. Season with salt and pepper. Serve fillets topped with tomato mixture.

Nutrition

Per Serving: 340 calories; protein 34.1g; carbohydrates 20.9g; fat 13.4g; cholesterol 69.8mg; sodium 604.4mg.

Tuna, Noodles, Pickles and Cheese

Prep:

10 mins

Cook:

10 mins

Total:

20 mins

Servings:

4

Yield:

4 servings

Ingredients

8 ounces uncooked elbow macaroni

6 ounces Colby-Jack cheese, cubed

½ cup light mayonnaise

2 dill pickles, chopped

½ teaspoon prepared yellow mustard

1 teaspoon dill pickle juice

1 (5 ounce) can albacore tuna in water, drained and flaked

Directions

1

Bring a saucepan of lightly salted water to a boil. Add the macaroni, and cook until tender, about 7 minutes. Rinse under cold running water, then drain well and pat lightly with paper towels.

2

In a large bowl, stir together the macaroni, pickles, cheese, tuna, mayonnaise and mustard. Season with a splash of pickle juice, salt and pepper. Cover, and refrigerate for at least 30 minutes before serving.

Nutrition

Per Serving: 491 calories; protein 26.3g; carbohydrates 55.4g; fat 18g; cholesterol 55.3mg; sodium 1611.2mg.

Tuna Stuffed Avocado

Prep:

20 mins

Total:

20 mins

Servings:

4

Yield:

4 servings

Ingredients

1 (12 ounce) can solid white tuna packed in water, drained
1 pinch garlic salt
1 tablespoon mayonnaise
½ red bell pepper, chopped
1 dash balsamic vinegar
black pepper to taste
2 ripe avocados, halved and pitted
3 green onions, thinly sliced, plus additional for garnish

Directions

1

Stir together tuna, mayonnaise, green onions, red pepper, and balsamic vinegar in a bowl. Season with pepper and garlic salt, then pack the avocado halves with the tuna mixture. Garnish with reserved green onions and a dash of black pepper before serving.

Nutrition

Per Serving: 294 calories; protein 23.9g; carbohydrates 11g; fat 18.2g; cholesterol 26.5mg; sodium 154.1mg.

Tuna-Stuffed Zucchini

Prep:

25 mins

Cook:

25 mins

Total:

50 mins

Servings:

6

Yield:

6 stuffed zucchini halves

Ingredients

3 zucchini, ends trimmed

¼ onion, grated

1 egg, beaten

salt and ground black pepper to taste

1 tablespoon olive oil

4 (3 ounce) cans tuna, drained and flaked

1 cup dry bread crumbs

Directions

1

Fill a large pot with salted water, place the zucchini into the pot, and boil over medium heat for about 5 minutes to soften. Remove the zucchini, slice in half lengthwise, and allow to cool.

2

Preheat oven to 350 degrees F. Lightly grease a 9x13-inch baking dish.

3

Scoop out the flesh from the zucchini halves, leaving a 1/2-inch shell. Set aside the scooped out flesh in a bowl.

4

Place the zucchini flesh into a bowl and mash well. Mix in the tuna, onion, tomato, bread crumbs, egg, salt, and black pepper. Lightly stuff the zucchini shells with the tuna mixture. Drizzle about 1/2 teaspoon of olive oil over each stuffed zucchini half.

5

Bake in the preheated oven until the tops are slightly browned, 20 to 25 minutes.

Nutrition

Per Serving: 193 calories; protein 19.4g; carbohydrates 18.2g; fat 4.7g; cholesterol 48mg; sodium 209.1mg.

Sticky Peanut Zoodles

Prep:

10 mins

Cook:

10 mins

Total:

20 mins

Servings:

1

Yield:

1 serving

Ingredients

1 medium zucchini, spiralized

¼ cup chopped peanuts

1 splash olive oil

2 cloves garlic, minced

1 tablespoon soy sauce

1 teaspoon brown sugar

1 pinch red pepper flakes

3 green onions, sliced

½ red bell pepper, thinly sliced

Directions

1

Heat a skillet over medium-high heat. Saute zucchini noodles in the hot pan for 4 minutes. Transfer to a metal colander and let drain in the sink.

2

Heat olive oil in the same pan over medium-low heat. Saute green onions and garlic in the hot oil, 2 to 3 minutes. Add soy sauce, brown sugar, and red pepper flakes. Let simmer until sauce is reduced and thick, about 5 minutes. Turn off heat.

3

Squeeze moisture out of zoodles in the colander. Toss into sticky sauce to coat. Serve topped with chopped peanuts and bell pepper.

Nutrition

Per Serving: 360 calories; protein 13.9g; carbohydrates 29.6g; fat 24g; sodium 1230.6mg.

Cauliflower Rice

Prep:

10 mins

Cook:

20 mins

Total:

30 mins

Servings:

4

Yield:

4 servings

Ingredients

1 head cauliflower, cut into florets

2 teaspoons chopped fresh chives

¼ teaspoon garlic powder

2 teaspoons chopped fresh parsley

salt and ground black pepper to taste

¼ teaspoon onion powder

Directions

1

Place a steamer insert into a pot and fill with water to just below the bottom of the steamer. Bring water to a boil. Add cauliflower, cover, and steam until fork-tender, 10 to 15 minutes.

2

Remove cauliflower and steamer from the pot. Drain all water and return cauliflower to the empty pot. Add chives, parsley, garlic powder, and onion powder.

3

Set pot over medium-low heat. Mash cauliflower with a potato masher to the consistency of rice grains. Stir until excess moisture evaporates and the 'rice' appears fluffy, 6 to 7 minutes. Season with salt and pepper.

Nutrition

Per Serving: 37 calories; protein 2.9g; carbohydrates 7.9g; fat 0.2g; sodium 82.4mg.

Shirataki Noodles

Prep:

10 mins

Cook:

25 mins

Total:

35 mins

Servings:

3

Yield:

3 servings

Ingredients

2 (8 ounce) packages shirataki noodles, drained and rinsed

1 tablespoon olive oil

2 cloves garlic, minced

¼ teaspoon red pepper flakes

12 ounces raw shrimp, peeled and deveined

¼ teaspoon salt

⅛ teaspoon ground black pepper

1 tablespoon minced shallot

3 tablespoons fresh lemon juice

2 tablespoons butter

1 tablespoon chopped fresh parsley

3 tablespoons dry white wine

Directions

1

Cover shirataki noodles with water and bring to a boil. Boil for 5 minutes. Drain.

2
Return drained noodles to the saucepan and cook over medium heat to remove any excess moisture, 5 to 6 minutes. Remove from heat and set aside.

3
Drizzle olive oil into a large skillet over medium heat. Add shallot and stir until translucent, 2 to 3 minutes. Take care not to burn. Add garlic and red pepper flakes; stir for 1 minute. Add shrimp and cook for 2 to 3 minutes per side, taking care not to overcook. Season with salt and pepper.

4
Transfer shrimp to a bowl, reserving pan drippings in the skillet. Whisk lemon juice and white wine into the skillet. Add butter and cook until fully incorporated and sauce begins to thicken slightly, 3 to 4 minutes.

5
Return shrimp to the skillet. Add noodles. Sprinkle with parsley and toss to combine.

Nutrition
Per Serving: 224 calories; protein 19g; carbohydrates 6.8g; fat 13.2g; cholesterol 190.7mg; sodium 461.4mg.

Italian Turkey Pasta Skillet

Prep:

15 mins

Cook:

15 mins

Total:

30 mins

Servings:

6

Yield:

6 servings

Ingredients

½ (16 ounce) package whole-wheat spaghetti

olive oil

1 cup shredded mozzarella cheese

1 green bell pepper, chopped

1 pound cubed cooked turkey

1 (26 ounce) jar spaghetti sauce

1 small red onion, thinly sliced

Directions

1

Fill a large pot with lightly salted water and bring to a rolling boil over high heat. Once the water is boiling, stir in the spaghetti, and return to a boil. Cook the pasta uncovered, stirring occasionally, until the pasta has cooked through, but is still firm to the bite, about 12 minutes. Drain well in a colander set in the sink.

2

Meanwhile, heat the olive oil in a large saucepan or Dutch oven over medium heat. Stir in the onion and green pepper. Cook and stir until the onion has softened and turned translucent, about 5 minutes. Stir in the turkey and spaghetti sauce. Bring to a simmer over medium-high heat, then cover, and reduce heat to medium-low. Cook until the sauce is hot.

3

Once the spaghetti has been cooked and drained, stir it into the hot sauce along with the mozzarella cheese. Stir until the cheese melts, then serve.

Nutrition

Per Serving: 442 calories; protein 34.8g; carbohydrates 47.6g; fat 12.8g; cholesterol 72mg; sodium 671.1mg.

Hot Sausage Pot

Prep:

30 mins

Cook:

1 hr

Total:

1 hr 30 mins

Servings:

6

Yield:

6 servings

Ingredients

1 (16 ounce) package spicy ground pork sausage
1 (12 fluid ounce) can beer
2 cups chicken broth
6 large potatoes, peeled and chopped
1 medium red bell pepper, chopped
1 medium yellow bell pepper, chopped
1 large sweet onion, chopped
1 large red onion, chopped
1 jalapeno pepper, finely chopped
1 medium green bell pepper, chopped
1 habanero pepper, seeded and chopped
¼ cup chopped green onions
2 cloves garlic, peeled and chopped
salt and pepper to taste
1 red chile peppers, seeded and chopped

Directions

1

Preheat oven to 350 degrees F.

2

In a large, deep skillet over medium high heat, cook sausage in the beer until evenly browned. Drain, and set aside.

3

In a large baking dish, mix sausage, potatoes, green bell pepper, red bell pepper, yellow bell pepper, sweet onion, red onion, jalapeno pepper, habanero pepper, red chile pepper, green onions, and garlic. Season with salt and pepper. Stir in chicken broth.

4

Cover, and bake in the preheated oven 1 hour, or until all vegetables are tender.

Nutrition

Per Serving: 668 calories; protein 18g; carbohydrates 76.9g; fat 31.1g; cholesterol 51.5mg; sodium 535.1mg.

Zucchini Caprese

Prep:

10 mins

Cook:

10 mins

Total:

20 mins

Servings:

2

Yield:

2 servings

Ingredients

1 tablespoon olive oil
2 roma (plum) tomatoes, diced
½ onion, chopped
2 cloves garlic, minced
salt and ground black pepper to taste
2 tablespoons chopped fresh basil
¼ cup shredded mozzarella cheese
1 zucchini, chopped

Directions

1

Heat olive oil in a skillet over medium heat. Cook and stir onion and garlic in hot oil until onion is translucent, 4 to 5 minutes; season with salt and pepper.

2

Stir zucchini and basil into the onion mixture; cook and stir until zucchini is soft, about 5 minutes. Add tomatoes and mozzarella cheese; cook and stir until the cheese melts, about 2 minutes.

Nutrition

Per Serving: 150 calories; protein 6.1g; carbohydrates 12.5g; fat 9.4g; cholesterol 9mg; sodium 103.4mg.

Catalan Shrimo with Mushrooms

Prep:

25 mins

Cook:

34 mins

Total:

59 mins

Servings:

6

Yield:

6 servings

Ingredients

1 (16 ounce) package angel hair pasta

¼ cup chopped scallions

½ cup butter

3 white mushrooms, sliced

2 cloves garlic, minced

½ cup dry white wine

½ cup chicken broth

½ (10 ounce) can stewed tomatoes

¼ cup finely chopped onion

2 tablespoons chopped fresh parsley

2 ounces all-purpose flour

1 pound large shrimp, peeled and deveined

1 pinch salt and ground black pepper to taste

Directions

1

Bring a large pot of lightly salted water to a boil. Cook angel hair pasta in the boiling water, stirring occasionally, until tender yet firm to the bite, 4 to 5 minutes. Drain.

2

Melt butter in a skillet over medium-high heat. Saute mushrooms, onion, scallions, and garlic until onions are translucent, about 5 minutes. Add wine, broth, tomatoes, and parsley. Bring sauce to a boil. Stir and reduce heat to low. Simmer, covered, for 10 minutes.

3

Place shrimp and flour in a resealable plastic bag; shake and mix until shrimp is well coated. Stir shrimp into the scampi. Cook until shrimp are opaque, about 5 minutes. Pour sauce and shrimp over the pasta; squeeze lemon juice on top. Season with salt and pepper.

Nutrition

Per Serving: 473 calories; protein 22.2g; carbohydrates 52.2g; fat 18.2g; cholesterol 155.7mg; sodium 476.3mg.

Pasta Primavera

Prep:

20 mins

Cook:

20 mins

Total:

40 mins

Servings:

4

Yield:

4 servings

Ingredients

2 cups whole grain penne pasta

1 tablespoon olive oil

⅛ teaspoon red pepper flakes

½ cup chopped onion

1 pound fresh asparagus, trimmed and cut into 2-inch pieces

2 cups sliced fresh mushrooms

2 cups cherry tomatoes, halved

½ cup shredded carrot

2 cloves garlic, minced

1 tablespoon chopped fresh oregano

½ teaspoon ground black pepper

1 small yellow summer squash, halved lengthwise and sliced

¼ teaspoon salt

½ cup freshly grated Parmesan cheese

Lemon wedges

Directions

1

Bring a large pot of lightly salted water to a boil. Add penne and cook, stirring occasionally, until tender yet firm to the bite, about 11 minutes.

2

Meanwhile, heat oil in an extra-large skillet over medium-high heat. Add onion; cook until softened, 2 to 3 minutes. Add asparagus, mushrooms, and squash; cook until just tender, about 5 minutes. Add tomatoes, carrot, garlic, oregano, black pepper, salt, and red pepper flakes; cook until tomatoes begin to soften, about 1 minute.

3

Drain penne; stir into vegetable mixture along with 1/4 cup Parmesan cheese. Top servings with remaining cheese and serve with lemon wedges.

Nutrition

Per Serving: 281 calories; protein 15.8g; carbohydrates 41.5g; fat 7.7g; cholesterol 8.8mg; sodium 337.6mg

Pork Goulash

Prep:

25 mins

Cook:

25 mins

Total:

50 mins

Servings:

8

Yield:

8 servings

Ingredients

1 pound macaroni

1 ½ pounds lean ground beef

1 small yellow onion, diced

1 green bell pepper, diced

1 cup sliced mushrooms

1 (8 ounce) can peas, drained

1 (14.5 ounce) can stewed tomatoes, cut in half and drained

1 (14.5 ounce) can crushed tomatoes

4 (6 ounce) cans tomato paste

2 (15 ounce) cans tomato sauce

24 fluid ounces water

1 tablespoon chopped garlic

1 tablespoon dried parsley

1 teaspoon salt

1 teaspoon black pepper

1 tablespoon grated Parmesan cheese

⅛ teaspoon white sugar

1 (8.75 ounce) can whole kernel corn, drained

Directions

1

Bring a large pot of lightly salted water to a boil. Add macaroni and cook for 9 to 10 minutes or until al dente; drain.

2

In a large saucepan, brown the ground beef with the onion, green pepper, and mushrooms; drain. Add corn, peas, stewed tomatoes, crushed tomatoes, tomato paste, tomato sauce, and water. Stir and bring to boil over medium heat. Mix in

, parmesan cheese, parsley, salt, pepper, sugar and simmer for 20 to 25 minutes.

3

Mix together cooked macaroni and meat sauce. Serve hot or refrigerate for later.

Nutrition

Per Serving: 560 calories; protein 31.2g; carbohydrates 81.4g; fat 14.4g; cholesterol 52mg; sodium 1925.9mg.

Oven-Roasted Tri-Tip

Prep:

5 mins

Cook:

30 mins

Additional:

2 hrs 15 mins

Total:

2 hrs 50 mins

Servings:

8

Yield:

8 servings

Ingredients

1 (2 pound) beef tri-tip roast

¼ cup soy sauce

1 onion, cut into wedges

2 teaspoons ground cumin

¼ cup vegetable oil

1 teaspoon ground black pepper

1 teaspoon crushed garlic

Directions

1

Toss tri-tip with oil, soy sauce, onion, cumin, garlic, and pepper. Marinate in the refrigerator for 2 hours, or up to 24 hours. Let rest at room temperature while preheating the oven.

2

Preheat the oven to 425 degrees F.

3

Place tri-tip in a shallow roasting pan, preferably on a rack. Remove onions from marinade and place around the beef.

4

Roast in the preheated oven until internal temperature reaches 135 degrees F for medium-rare or 150 degrees F for medium, 30 to 45 minutes.

5

Allow to rest at least 15 minutes before slicing against the grain.

Nutrition

Per Serving: 292 calories; protein 31.3g; carbohydrates 3.8g; fat 16.3g; cholesterol 105.4mg; sodium 492.8mg.

CHAPTER 6: APPETIZER, SNACKS & SIDE DISHES

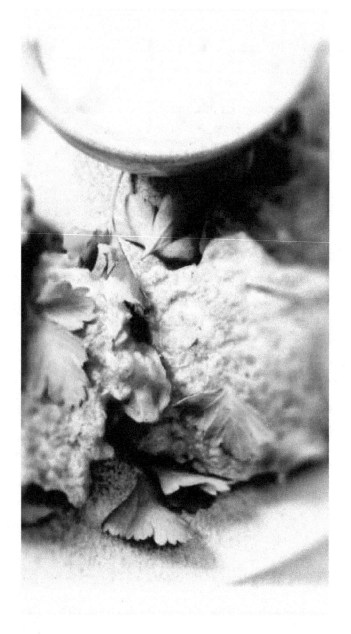

Pickled Shallots

Prep:

5 mins

Cook:

10 mins

Total:

15 mins

Servings:

4

Yield:

4 servings

Ingredients

3 tablespoons butter
2 tablespoons liquid honey
1 pound shallots, peeled and quartered
4 sprigs fresh thyme, chopped
salt and pepper to taste
7 tablespoons balsamic vinegar

Directions

1

Melt butter in a medium skillet over medium heat; stir in honey and shallots. Season with thyme, salt, and pepper and cook until lightly browned, 2 to 3 minutes. Turn shallots to brown evenly.

2

Pour balsamic vinegar into the skillet with the shallots. Reduce heat to low and simmer until shallots are soft, about 7 minutes.

3

Serve warm or store shallots in the refrigerator in a sealed container until chilled.

Nutrition

Per Serving: 236 calories; protein 4.6g; carbohydrates 38.7g; fat 9.3g; cholesterol 22.9mg; sodium 123.4mg.

Cauliflower Fritters

Prep:

10 mins

Cook:

10 mins

Total:

20 mins

Servings:

6

Yield:

6 servings

Ingredients

6 cups cauliflower florets

½ cup all-purpose flour

3 extra large eggs

1 teaspoon baking powder

1 (.7 ounce) package dry Italian-style salad dressing mix

½ cup olive oil for frying, or as needed

Directions

1

Process cauliflower in a food processor finely minced; transfer to a large bowl.

2

Stir flour, eggs, baking powder, and Italian dressing mix into cauliflower.

3

Heat enough olive oil to cover the bottom of a frying pan over medium heat.

4

Drop heaping tablespoons of cauliflower mixture into the hot oil; fry until golden brown, about 3 minutes per side.

Nutrition

Per Serving: 129 calories; protein 6.7g; carbohydrates 15.3g; fat 4.9g; cholesterol 107.9mg; sodium 682.2mg.

Carrot and Parsnip Puree

Prep:

15 mins

Cook:

35 mins

Total:

50 mins

Servings:

4

Yield:

4 servings

Ingredients

1 tablespoon butter, or to taste
1 pound carrots, peeled and finely chopped
⅔ pound parsnips, peeled and chopped
½ onion, chopped
½ cup water
½ cup chicken stock
2 green onions, thinly sliced
salt and ground black pepper to taste

Directions

1

Melt 1 tablespoon butter in a saucepan over medium heat. Stir carrots, parsnips, onion, water, chicken stock, and green onion with the butter; bring to a boil, reduce heat to low, place a cover on the saucepan, and cook until the vegetables are very tender, about 30 minutes.

2

Blend the vegetable mixture in the saucepan with an immersion blender; season with salt and pepper. Add more butter, to your taste.

Nutrition

Per Serving: 145 calories; protein 2.8g; carbohydrates 27.8g; fat 3.5g; cholesterol 8.1mg; sodium 162.4mg.

Hemp Seed Oatmeal

Prep:

5 mins

Cook:

15 mins

Total:

20 mins

Servings:

2

Yield:

2 servings

Ingredients

1 cup water
1 cup apple cider
1 cup rolled oats
1 Granny Smith apple, diced
1 teaspoon ground cinnamon
½ teaspoon vanilla extract
¼ cup hemp milk
¼ cup hemp seeds

Directions

1

Bring water and apple cider to a boil in a medium saucepan. Stir in oats, reduce heat to low, and cook, stirring occasionally, for 3 minutes. Add apple, cinnamon, and vanilla extract. Cook, stirring gently, until tender, about 3 minutes more.

2

Remove oatmeal from heat; add hemp milk and hemp seeds. Stir and serve.

Green Beans and Ham

Prep:

20 mins

Cook:

25 mins

Total:

45 mins

Servings:

8

Yield:

8 servings

Ingredients

1 (2 pound) ham steak, cut into 1-inch pieces
1 ½ pounds red new potatoes, halved
1 pound fresh green beans, trimmed and halved
1 small onion, coarsely chopped
½ cup butter
water to cover
salt and ground black pepper to taste

Directions

1

Place ham steak, potatoes, green beans, onion, and butter in a large pot
with just enough water to cover. Season with salt and pepper; bring to
a boil. Reduce heat to medium-low and simmer until potatoes are
tender, about 20 minutes.

Nutrition

Per Serving: 327 calories; protein 25.2g; carbohydrates 19.7g; fat 16.5g; cholesterol 81.6mg; sodium 1553.8mg.

Chicken Paprika

Prep:

20 mins

Cook:

20 mins

Total:

40 mins

Servings:

12

Yield:

12 servings

Ingredients

⅓ cup all-purpose flour

2 tablespoons paprika

1 teaspoon salt

1 pinch ground black pepper

6 skinless, boneless chicken breast halves, cut into bite-size pieces

2 tablespoons vegetable oil

1 onion, chopped

4 cloves garlic, minced

1 cup chicken stock

2 tablespoons tomato paste

1 ½ cups sour cream

1 tablespoon paprika

1 teaspoon cornstarch

Directions

1

Mix flour, 2 tablespoons paprika, salt, and pepper on a shallow plate. Dip chicken pieces in mixture to coat.

2

Heat vegetable oil in a heavy skillet over medium heat. Cook and stir chicken in hot oil until browned completely, about 5 minutes. Remove chicken with a slotted spoon to a bowl, reserving oil and drippings in skillet.

3

Cook and stir onion and garlic in the reserved drippings until tender, about 5 minutes. Return chicken to the skillet. Pour chicken stock over the chicken mixture. Stir tomato paste into the chicken stock until integrated completely.

4

Bring the chicken stock to a boil, reduce heat to medium-low, place a cover on the skillet, and cook at a simmer until the chicken is cooked through, 5 to 8 minutes.

5

Whisk sour cream, 1 teaspoon paprika, and cornstarch together in a small bowl; stir into the chicken mixture and cook until hot, 2 to 3 minutes.

Nutrition

Per Serving: 170 calories; protein 13g; carbohydrates 7.8g; fat 9.8g; cholesterol 42mg; sodium 313.1mg.

Sweet and Spicy Dipping Sauce

Prep:

5 mins

Cook:

15 mins

Additional:

15 mins

Total:

35 mins

Servings:

16

Yield:

1 cup

Ingredients

½ cup rice wine vinegar
½ cup white sugar
2 teaspoons salt
1 tablespoon chili garlic sauce (such as Lee Kum Kee®)

Directions

1

Stir the vinegar and sugar together in a small saucepan over medium heat until the sugar dissolves completely, 7 to 10 minutes; add the salt, reduce heat to low, and simmer until the mixture thickens slightly, about 5 minutes. Remove from heat and stir the chili garlic sauce into the mixture. Allow to cool slightly before serving.

Nutrition

Per Serving: 25 calories; carbohydrates 6.3g; sodium 330.4mg.

Chili Avocado-Chimichurri Sauce

Prep:

10 mins

Total:

10 mins

Servings:

6

Yield:

6 servings

Ingredients

3 small avocados, flesh removed

½ white onion, cut into large chunks

½ bunch cilantro

½ bunch parsley

1 jalapeno pepper, seeded

1 lime, juiced

3 tablespoons white balsamic vinegar

3 cloves garlic, minced

salt and ground black pepper to taste

¼ cup extra-virgin olive oil

Directions

1

Blend avocado, white onion, cilantro, parsley, jalapeno pepper, lime juice, white balsamic vinegar, garlic, salt, and pepper in a blender until everything is thoroughly chopped. Stream olive oil into the avocado mixture while blending until the mixture is smooth and creamy.

Nutrition

Per Serving: 236 calories; protein 2.2g; carbohydrates 10.9g; fat 21.9g; sodium 13.6mg.

All Seed Flapjacks

Prep:

15 mins

Cook:

15 mins

Total:

30 mins

Servings:

8

Yield:

8 servings

Ingredients

½ cup butter

3 tablespoons white sugar

2 tablespoons golden syrup

2 cups rolled oats

5 tablespoons raisins (Optional)

1 (5 ounce) milk chocolate, melted (Optional)

Directions

1

Preheat the oven to 350 degrees F (175 degrees C). Lightly butter a baking pan.

2

Combine butter, sugar, and golden syrup in a saucepan over low heat. Mix until butter has melted and sugar has dissolved. Remove from heat. Add 2 cups oats and raisins. Mix until oats are well coated. Pour mixture into the prepared pan; flatten down with the back of a spoon.

3

Bake in the preheated oven until golden brown on top, 10 to 20 minutes. Let flapjack cool.

4

Melt chocolate in a microwave-safe glass or ceramic bowl in 15-second intervals, stirring after each interval, 1 to 3 minutes. Pour over the cooled flapjack. Let cool until chocolate is set.

Nutrition

Per Serving: 330 calories; protein 4.4g; carbohydrates 38.5g; fat 18.4g; cholesterol 34.8mg; sodium 101.6mg.

Herbie's Home Fries

Prep:

30 mins

Cook:

30 mins

Total:

1 hr

Servings:

4

Yield:

4 servings

Ingredients

4 large Yukon Gold potatoes
6 tablespoons butter
1 large sweet onion, diced
1 medium green bell pepper, diced
1 clove garlic, crushed
1 tablespoon Hungarian sweet paprika
salt and pepper to taste

Directions

1

Bring a large pot of salted water to a boil. Add potatoes, and cook until tender but still firm, about 15 minutes. Drain, cool and chop.

2

Melt 4 tablespoons butter in a medium saucepan over medium heat. Stir in onion, green bell pepper and garlic, and cook until tender, 5 to 10 minutes.

3

Mix potatoes and remaining butter into the saucepan. Season with paprika, salt and pepper. Cook and stir until well mixed and tender, 15 to 20 minutes. Cover while cooking if moist potatoes are preferred.

Nutrition

Per Serving: 325 calories; protein 5g; carbohydrates 39.2g; fat 17.8g; cholesterol 45.8mg; sodium 136.8mg.

Mixed Seed Crackers

Prep:

5 mins

Additional:

3 hrs

Total:

3 hrs 5 mins

Servings:

15

Yield:

15 servings

Ingredients

1 (1 ounce) package ranch dressing mix

1 ½ cups vegetable oil

1 (16 ounce) package saltine crackers

Directions

1

Place ranch dressing mix and vegetable oil in a 2-gallon resealable bag; seal and shake until well combined. Add crackers and shake until crackers are fully coated. Set aside for 3 hours to allow crackers to absorb coating, shaking bag every 1/2 hour.

Nutrition

Per Serving: 325 calories; protein 2.8g; carbohydrates 22.1g; fat 25.2g; sodium 450.8mg.

Keto Snickerdoodles

Prep:

15 mins

Cook:

35 mins

Total:

50 mins

Servings:

20

Yield:

4 mini loaves

Ingredients

Bread:

2 cups white sugar

1 cup butter, softened

2 teaspoons ground cinnamon

½ teaspoon salt

3 eggs

¾ cup sour cream

1 teaspoon vanilla extract

2 ½ cups all-purpose flour

1 teaspoon baking powder

1 (10 ounce) package cinnamon chips (such as HERSHEY'S®)

Topping:

3 tablespoons white sugar

3 teaspoons ground cinnamon

Directions

1

Preheat the oven to 350 degrees F (175 degrees C). Grease 4 mini loaf pans.

2

Cream together sugar, butter, cinnamon, and salt with an electric mixer until fluffy, about 5 minutes. Add eggs and mix well. Mix in sour cream and vanilla until combined.

3

Combine flour and baking powder in a separate bowl. Pour into egg mixture and mix well. Stir cinnamon chips into batter. Spoon batter into 4 mini loaf pans until 2/3 full.

4

Mix 3 tablespoons sugar and cinnamon together in a small bowl. Sprinkle topping over the batter in each loaf pan.

5

Bake in the preheated oven until a toothpick inserted into the centers come out clean, 35 to 38 minutes. Let cool completely before removing from the pans.

Nutrition

Per Serving: 329 calories; protein 4g; carbohydrates 43.3g; fat 15.9g; cholesterol 56.7mg; sodium 193.5mg.

Snakes in a Blanket

Prep:

15 mins

Cook:

13 mins

Total:

28 mins

Servings:

8

Yield:

8 servings

Ingredients

1 (10 ounce) can refrigerated crescent roll dough

1 tablespoon olive oil (Optional)

4 slices provolone cheese, halved

4 slices Swiss cheese, halved

4 slices mozzarella cheese, halved

8 asparagus spears, trimmed and cut in half

2 tablespoons olive oil, for drizzling (Optional)

1 tablespoon dried Italian seasoning (Optional)

Directions

1

Preheat oven to 350 degrees F (175 degrees C). Lightly grease a baking sheet.

2

Unroll and separate dough into 8 triangles; place on a lightly floured surface. Using 1 tablespoon of olive oil, lightly brush the top of each dough triangle. Place one piece of provolone cheese, Swiss cheese and mozzarella cheese on the wide end of each triangle. Put one piece of asparagus on top of the cheese. Roll each dough triangle around the cheese and asparagus toward the point and press to secure. Arrange on a baking sheet at least 2 inches apart.

3

Bake in preheated oven until lightly brown, 13 to 18 minutes. Remove from the baking sheet to cool on wire racks. If desired, drizzle with 2 tablespoons olive oil and sprinkle with Italian seasoning.

Nutrition

Per Serving: 299 calories; protein 11.8g; carbohydrates 15.8g; fat 20.6g; cholesterol 25.3mg; sodium 500mg.

CHAPTER 7: VEGAN & VEGETARIAN

Brussels Sprouts Caesar

Prep:

20 mins

Cook:

20 mins

Total:

40 mins

Servings:

6

Yield:

6 servings

Ingredients

2 (16 ounce) packages Brussels sprouts

¼ cup olive oil, divided

2 teaspoons smoked paprika, divided

¼ teaspoon sea salt

¼ cup heavy whipping cream

1 tablespoon red wine vinegar

1 lemon, zested and juiced

2 cloves garlic, minced

1 teaspoon brown mustard

3 tablespoons grated Parmesan cheese

Directions

1

Preheat oven to 425 degrees F.

2

Trim stems off Brussels sprouts. Quarter large sprouts lengthwise; halve small ones. Rinse and dry completely.

3

Toss sprouts in a bowl with 1 tablespoon olive oil and 1 teaspoon paprika. Spread out on a baking sheet and sprinkle with sea salt.

4

Bake in the preheated oven for 20 minutes, removing loose leaves after 5 minutes and turning whole sprouts every 5 minutes.

5

Whisk remaining 3 tablespoons olive oil, remaining 1 teaspoon paprika, heavy cream, Parmesan cheese, red wine vinegar, lemon zest and juice, garlic, and brown mustard together in a bowl.

6

Transfer whole sprouts and any loose leaves to a bowl; pour in cream mixture and toss to combine.

Nutrition

Per Serving: 199 calories; protein 6.7g; carbohydrates 16.9g; fat 14g; cholesterol 15.8mg; sodium 165.1mg.

Beanie-Weenie

Prep:

15 mins

Cook:

30 mins

Total:

45 mins

Servings:

6

Yield:

6 servings

Ingredients

1 (16 ounce) package hot dogs , cut into 1/4-inch slices

⅔ cup ketchup

1 ½ teaspoons garlic powder

1 (28 ounce) can baked beans with pork

1 tablespoon chopped fresh parsley

2 tablespoons cider vinegar

¼ cup Worcestershire sauce

Directions

1

In a large skillet, combine the hot dogs, baked beans, ketchup, cider vinegar, Worcestershire sauce, garlic powder and parsley. Mix to blend, and bring to a boil. Turn heat to low, cover, and simmer for 25 to 30 minutes, stirring occasionally.

Nutrition

Per Serving: 433 calories; protein 16g; carbohydrates 40.5g; fat 24.1g; cholesterol 48.9mg; sodium 1702.8mg.

Kapusta

Prep:

20 mins

Cook:

1 hr 10 mins

Total:

1 hr 30 mins

Servings:

6

Yield:

6 servings

Ingredients

6 tablespoons butter, divided
½ teaspoon white sugar
½ teaspoon dried thyme
2 onions, chopped
1 ½ cups sliced mushrooms
¼ medium head cabbage, thinly sliced
1 (32 ounce) jar sauerkraut, drained and pressed
1 large portobello mushrooms, sliced
salt and pepper to taste

Directions

1

Preheat oven to 350 degrees F.

2

Heat 4 tablespoons of butter over medium heat; saute onions and mushrooms until tender.

3

In a medium saucepan over high heat, boil cabbage for 10 minutes.

4

In a 9 x 13 inch baking dish combine onions, mushrooms, cabbage, sauerkraut, sugar, thyme, salt and pepper; mix well. Dot remaining 2 tablespoons butter on top. Cover.

5

Bake in preheated oven for 1 hour, stirring every 20 minutes.

Nutrition

Per Serving: 151 calories; protein 2.6g; carbohydrates 11g; fat 11.8g; cholesterol 30.5mg; sodium 760.5mg.

Pasta with Alfredo Sauce

Prep:

10 mins

Cook:

10 mins

Total:

20 mins

Servings:

4

Yield:

4 servings

Ingredients

¼ cup butter

1 ½ cups freshly grated Parmesan cheese

¼ cup chopped fresh parsley

1 cup heavy cream

1 clove garlic, crushed

Directions

1

Melt butter in a medium saucepan over medium low heat. Add cream and simmer for 5 minutes, then add garlic and cheese and whisk quickly, heating through. Stir in parsley and serve.

Nutrition

Per Serving: 439 calories; protein 13g; carbohydrates 3.4g; fat 42.1g; cholesterol 138.4mg; sodium 565.3mg.

Kohlrabi with Garlic-Mushroom Sauce

Prep:

10 mins

Cook:

35 mins

Total:

45 mins

Servings:

4

Yield:

4 servings

Ingredients

6 kohlrabi, peeled
2 tablespoons butter
2 tablespoons heavy whipping cream
salt to taste
2 tablespoons all-purpose flour
ground white pepper to taste
1 bunch flat-leaf parsley, finely chopped

Directions

1

Place a steamer insert into a saucepan and fill with water to just below the bottom of the steamer. Bring water to a boil. Add kohlrabi, cover, and steam until tender, 20 to 25 minutes. Reserve cooking water.

2

Melt butter in a saucepan over medium-low heat. Whisk in flour and stir until the mixture becomes paste-like and light golden brown, about 5 minutes. Gradually whisk the kohlrabi cooking water into the flour mixture, and bring to a simmer over medium heat. Cook and stir until thickened, about 6 minutes. Add parsley. Stir in heavy cream. Add kohlrabi; season with salt and pepper.

Nutrition

Per Serving: 178 calories; protein 6.2g; carbohydrates 22.9g; fat 9g; cholesterol 25.5mg; sodium 151mg.

Keto Coleslaw

Prep:

15 mins

Total:

15 mins

Servings:

8

Yield:

8 servings

Ingredients

1 medium head cabbage, shredded

1 carrot

¼ cup vegetable oil

¼ cup vinegar

¼ cup white sugar

¼ onion, chopped

Directions

1

In a large bowl, combine cabbage, carrot, onion, vegetable oil, vinegar and sugar. Stir until the ingredients are well mixed. Chill in the refrigerator until serving.

Nutrition

Per Serving: 119 calories; protein 1.6g; carbohydrates 14g; fat 7g; sodium 26.8mg.

Vegetarian Borscht

Prep:

15 mins

Cook:

45 mins

Total:

1 hr

Servings:

6

Yield:

6 servings

Ingredients

3 tablespoons vinegar

2 tablespoons vegetable oil

1 onion, chopped

2 carrot, coarsely grated

8 cups water

¼ medium head cabbage, shredded

salt and pepper to taste

2 tablespoons tomato paste

2 tablespoons sour cream

2 small beets, peeled and coarsely grated

2 tablespoons chopped fresh dill

¾ cup dry yellow lentils

3 medium potatoes, peeled and diced

Directions

1

Combine beets and vinegar in a small frying pan over low heat. Cook, while stirring, until soft, about 15 minutes.

2

Heat oil in a large frying pan over low heat while beets are cooking. Add onion and stir for 2 minutes. Add carrots and cook, stirring occasionally, until soft, about 10 minutes. Set aside.

3

In the meantime, bring water to a simmer in a large saucepan. Add cabbage and lentils. Cook for 10 minutes. Add potatoes and cook for 10 minutes more. Stir in cooked beets and onion-carrot mixture. Season with salt and pepper. Add tomato paste and simmer until all vegetables are tender, about 10 minutes more. Serve with sour cream and dill.

Nutrition

Per Serving: 264 calories; protein 10.3g; carbohydrates 43.8g; fat 6.1g; cholesterol 2.1mg; sodium 134.7mg.

Keto Crunch Cereal

Servings:

12

Yield:

2 dozen

Ingredients

¼ cup peanut butter
3 ½ cups cornflakes cereal
2 cups butterscotch chips

Directions

1

Melt the butterscotch chips over low heat and add peanut butter.

2

Stir in cornflakes.

3

Drop on waxed paper and let cool.

Nutrition

Per Serving: 223 calories; protein 1.9g; carbohydrates 26.4g; fat 10.8g; sodium 114mg.

Pine Nut Macaroons

Servings:

60

Yield:

5 dozen

Ingredients

1 pound almond paste

4 egg whites

4 cups pine nuts

1 ¼ cups white sugar

Directions

1

Preheat oven to 350 degrees F. Grease cookie sheets.

2

Break almond paste into pieces and mix together with sugar, using your hands to crumble paste. In a separate bowl, separate the eggs and beat the whites into soft peaks. Slowly add to almond paste mixture and mix until just blended.

3

Place pine nuts into bowl. Roll dough into 1-inch balls and press into nuts. Coat evenly and place on cookie sheets about 1 inch apart.

4

Bake 15 to 17 minutes, until lightly golden. Let cool on cookie sheets for 5 minutes, then transfer to racks.

Nutrition

Per Serving: 103 calories; protein 3.1g; carbohydrates 9.1g; fat 6.7g; sodium 4.7mg.

Chocolate Salami

Prep:

20 mins

Additional:

8 hrs

Total:

8 hrs 20 mins

Servings:

18

Yield:

3 chocolate salami

Ingredients

½ cup raisins

1 tablespoon confectioners' sugar for dusting

¼ cup cognac

2 cups unsweetened cocoa powder

1 ½ cups melted butter

1 (14 ounce) can sweetened condensed milk

2 (7 ounce) packages plain tea biscuits, broken into small pieces

1 cup whole blanched almonds

Directions

1

Soak the raisins in the cognac in a small dish for 10 minutes. Combine the tea biscuits, almonds, and cocoa powder in a large mixing bowl. Pour the cognac and raisins into the mixture along with the butter and condensed milk. Mix well with your hands until a stiff, dark, and moist dough is formed.

2

Roll a double layer of plastic wrap onto a clean work surface and place one third of the dough into the center of it. Shape the dough into a log about 2 to 3 inches in diameter. Place log towards the end of the plastic wrap and start rolling the plastic tightly around the log. Twist the ends of the plastic like a candy wrapper and tuck them under the log. Repeat with remaining dough. Refrigerate overnight.

3

When ready to serve, use a small sieve to sprinkle the outside of the logs with confectioner's sugar, or, if you prefer, sprinkle the confectioner's sugar on a kitchen towel and roll the log on it. Slice with a sharp knife to serve.

Nutrition

Per Serving: 405 calories; protein 7.2g; carbohydrates 36.7g; fat 27.5g; cholesterol 48.1mg; sodium 323.1mg.

Vegetarian Meatballs

Prep:

15 mins

Cook:

1 hr 20 mins

Total:

1 hr 35 mins

Servings:

20

Yield:

100 small meatballs

Ingredients

4 cups shredded mozzarella cheese

1 ½ cups finely ground pecans

1 (1 ounce) package dry onion soup mix

22 fluid ounces milk

2 teaspoons celery salt

8 eggs

2 cups cracker crumbs

vegetable oil for frying

1 (10.75 ounce) can condensed cream of mushroom soup

Directions

1

Combine mozzarella cheese, eggs, cracker crumbs, pecans, onion soup mix, and celery salt in a large bowl. Form mixture into small meatballs.

2

Heat oil in a deep-fryer or large saucepan. Cook meatballs in batches until browned and crispy, about 5 minutes. Drain on a baking sheet lined paper towels.

3

Transfer meatballs to a large slow cooker. Cover with cream of mushroom soup. Use the empty can to measure and pour in milk. Cook on Low until flavors combine and soup mixture thickens, 30 minutes to 2 hours.

Nutrition

Per Serving: 246 calories; protein 11.1g; carbohydrates 14.4g; fat 16.3g; cholesterol 91.5mg; sodium 555.3mg.

Spinach Egg White Muffins

Prep:

10 mins

Cook:

20 mins

Total:

30 mins

Servings:

10

Yield:

10 mini muffins

Ingredients

cooking spray

2 (4 ounce) cartons liquid egg whites

1 (10 ounce) package frozen chopped spinach, thawed and drained

1 teaspoon hot sauce

1 teaspoon salt

6 ounces shredded reduced-fat sharp Cheddar cheese

½ teaspoon ground black pepper

Directions

1

Preheat the oven to 350 degrees F. Spray a muffin tin with cooking spray.

2

Mix egg whites, Cheddar cheese, spinach, hot sauce, salt, and pepper in a bowl. Ladle mixture into the muffin tin, filling each cup 3/4 the way full.

3

Bake in the preheated oven until a knife inserted in the center of a muffin comes out clean, 20 to 25 minutes. Serve warm or cooled.

Nutrition

Per Serving: 59 calories; protein 8.2g; carbohydrates 1.8g; fat 2.2g; cholesterol 3.8mg; sodium 405.1mg.

Vegetable Ratatouille

Servings:

8

Yield:

8 servings

Ingredients

2 onion, sliced into thin rings

1 bay leaf

2 tablespoons chopped fresh parsley

3 cloves garlic, minced

1 medium eggplant, cubed

2 zucchini, cubed

1 yellow bell pepper, diced

1 chopped red bell pepper

4 roma (plum) tomatoes, chopped

½ cup olive oil

2 medium yellow squash, cubed

2 green bell peppers, seeded and cubed

4 sprigs fresh thyme

salt and pepper to taste

Directions

1

Heat 1 1/2 tablespoon of the oil in a large pot over medium-low heat. Add the onions and garlic and cook until soft.

2

In a large skillet, heat 1 1/2 tablespoon of olive oil and saute the zucchini in batches until slightly browned on all sides. Remove the zucchini and place in the pot with the onions and garlic.

3

Saute all the remaining vegetables one batch at a time, adding 1 1/2 tablespoon olive oil to the skillet each time you add a new set of vegetables. Once each batch has been sauteed add them to the large pot as was done in   2.

4

Season with salt and pepper. Add the bay leaf and thyme and cover the pot. Cook over medium heat for 15 to 20 minutes.

5

Add the chopped tomatoes and parsley to the large pot, cook another 10-15 minutes. Stir occasionally.

6

Remove the bay leaf and adjust seasoning.

Nutrition

Per Serving: 191 calories; protein 3.2g; carbohydrates 15.9g; fat 14.1g; sodium 13.1mg.

Aromatic Chinese Cabbage

Prep:

15 mins

Cook:

10 mins

Total:

25 mins

Servings:

12

Yield:

12 servings

Ingredients

1 (3 ounce) package ramen noodles, crushed

1 bunch green onions, chopped

½ cup white sugar

½ cup vegetable oil

¼ cup cider vinegar

10 ounces cashew pieces

1 (16 ounce) package shredded coleslaw mix

1 tablespoon soy sauce

Directions

1

In a preheated 350 degree F oven, toast the crushed noodles and nuts until golden brown.

2

In a large bowl, combine the coleslaw, green onions, toasted ramen noodles and cashews.

3

To prepare the dressing, whisk together the sugar, oil, vinegar and soy sauce. Pour the dressing over the salad, toss and serve.

Nutrition

Per Serving: 291 calories; protein 4.6g; carbohydrates 22.8g; fat 21.3g; cholesterol 3mg; sodium 262.9mg.

Chives Cheese Bites

Prep:

15 mins

Cook:

25 mins

Additional:

1 hr

Total:

1 hr 40 mins

Servings:

54

Yield:

9 dozen

Ingredients

1 cup butter, softened

½ teaspoon pepper sauce (such as Frank's Red Hot®)

3 cups shredded sharp Cheddar cheese

½ teaspoon salt

¼ teaspoon garlic powder

2 cups crisp rice cereal

2 cups all-purpose flour

¼ cup chopped fresh chives

Directions

1

In a large bowl, mix together the softened butter and cheese until well blended. Stir in flour, chives, salt, hot pepper sauce and garlic powder until thoroughly mixed. Stir in cereal. Divide the mixture into four parts, and roll into 6 inch long logs. Wrap in plastic wrap, and refrigerate until firm, about 1 hour.

2

Preheat the oven to 325 degrees F. Unwrap the cheese logs, and slice into 1/4 inch thick rounds. Place on an ungreased cookie sheet.

3

Bake for 20 to 25 minutes in the preheated oven, until edges are crisp and slightly browned.

Nutrition
Per Serving: 82 calories; protein 2.5g; carbohydrates 4.5g; fat 6g; cholesterol 17.1mg; sodium 101.6mg.

Ethiopian-Style Peppers

Prep:

45 mins

Cook:

15 mins

Total:

1 hr

Servings:

6

Yield:

6 servings

Ingredients

6 large green bell peppers
3 tablespoons olive oil
1 ½ links of andouille sausage, diced
1 cup uncooked long-grain white rice
1 onion, diced
½ teaspoon dried oregano
1 tablespoon Creole seasoning
black pepper to taste
¾ pound shrimp, peeled and deveined
2 ½ cups chicken broth
1 (8 ounce) can tomato sauce
2 cloves garlic, minced

Directions

1

Preheat oven to 325 degrees F. Grease an 8x12 inch baking dish. Bring a large pot of water to a boil. Remove tops and seeds from peppers. Blanch in boiling water 3 minutes. Drain on paper towels.

2

Heat olive oil in a large, deep skillet over medium heat. Saute onion until translucent. Stir in garlic, and season with oregano, Creole seasoning and black pepper. Stir in shrimp and sausage, and cook until shrimp turns pink, 5 minutes. Stir in rice, and cook 1 minute. Pour in chicken broth and tomato sauce. Cook until thick, 15 to 20 minutes. Fill peppers with stuffing mixture, and place in baking dish.

3

Bake in preheated oven for 15 to 20 minutes, or until heated through. Serve with lemon wedges and hot sauce.

Nutrition

Per Serving: 307 calories; protein 17g; carbohydrates 39.9g; fat 9.6g; cholesterol 90.2mg; sodium 954.3mg.

Aloo Gobi

Prep:

15 mins

Cook:

1 hr

Total:

1 hr 15 mins

Servings:

6

Yield:

6 servings

Ingredients

½ cup vegetable oil

1 teaspoon sea salt

3 large potatoes, cubed

2 tablespoons Madras curry powder

3 large carrots, chopped

1 (10 ounce) package frozen peas

1 head cauliflower, cut into florets

Directions

1

Preheat the oven to 350 degrees F.

2

Mix oil, curry powder, and salt together in a small bowl.

3

Combine potatoes and carrots in a large bowl; pour 2/3 of the curry sauce on top. Mix to combine. Spread on a large, rimmed baking sheet.

4

Bake in the preheated oven for 30 minutes. Mix cauliflower with remaining curry sauce. Add to the baking sheet and continue baking for 20 minutes. Add peas; bake for 10 minutes more. Garnish with cilantro.

Nutrition

Per Serving: 385 calories; protein 8.7g; carbohydrates 48.5g; fat 19g; sodium 412.3mg.

Jambalaya

Prep:

20 mins

Cook:

1 hr 15 mins

Total:

1 hr 35 mins

Servings:

8

Yield:

8 servings

Ingredients

2 tablespoons canola oil

1 cup chopped celery

2 teaspoons minced garlic

1 large onion, chopped

1 large green bell pepper, chopped

1 (8 ounce) package sliced fresh mushrooms

1 (28 ounce) can diced tomatoes with juice

1 (19 ounce) can vegetarian hot dogs (such as Loma Linda® Big Franks), sliced

½ teaspoon dried thyme

2 (12.5 ounce) cans vegetarian fried chicken (such as FriChik®), chopped

1 cup vegetarian chicken-flavored broth

2 teaspoons dried parsley

2 teaspoons Cajun seasoning

1 teaspoon cayenne pepper

1 cup brown rice

2 teaspoons dried oregano

Directions

1

Preheat oven to 350 degrees F.

2

Heat canola oil in a large pan over medium heat; cook and stir onion, bell pepper, mushrooms, celery, and garlic until onion is tender and translucent, about 5 minutes. Add tomatoes, vegetarian hot dogs, vegetarian fried chicken, vegetarian chicken broth, brown rice, oregano, parsley, Cajun seasoning, cayenne pepper, and thyme. Cook and stir until boiling, about 10 minutes. Transfer mixture to a large baking dish.

3

Bake in preheated oven until rice is tender, about 1 hour.

Nutrition

Per Serving: 323 calories; protein 20.5g; carbohydrates 28.7g; fat 13.9g; sodium 652mg.

Eggplant Bolognese

Prep:

15 mins

Cook:

1 hr

Total:

1 hr 15 mins

Servings:

6

Yield:

6 servings

Ingredients

¼ cup olive oil, divided

3 links pork sausage, casings removed

1 small yellow onion, chopped

1 teaspoon dried parsley

1 teaspoon dried oregano

3 cloves garlic, minced

1 ½ teaspoons sea salt

¾ teaspoon freshly ground black pepper

1 (8 ounce) package sliced fresh mushrooms

1 (28 ounce) can crushed tomatoes

½ pound ground beef

2 pounds eggplant, peeled and chopped

1 (12 ounce) can petite diced tomatoes

1 ½ teaspoons dried basil

Directions

1

Heat 2 tablespoons olive oil in a large Dutch oven over medium heat; cook pork sausage, breaking it onto smaller pieces with a wooden spoon, until browned, about 5 minutes. Add ground beef; cook and stir until beef is browned and crumbly, about 5 minutes. Drain excess fat.

2

Pour remaining olive oil over sausage mixture; add eggplant, onion, garlic, salt, and black pepper. Cook and stir until lightly browned, about 10 minutes. Add mushrooms and continuing cooking until tender, about 5 minutes.

3

Mix crushed tomatoes, diced tomatoes, parsley, oregano, and basil into sausage mixture; bring to a boil. Cover Dutch oven, reduce heat to medium-low, and simmer for 30 minutes.

Nutrition

Per Serving: 282 calories; protein 14.1g; carbohydrates 19.2g; fat 17.7g; cholesterol 34.2mg; sodium 839.6mg.

Moroccan Chickpea Stew

Prep:

25 mins

Cook:

55 mins

Total:

1 hr 20 mins

Servings:

6

Yield:

6 servings

Ingredients

1 pint cherry tomatoes

3 cloves garlic, minced

3 tablespoons olive oil, divided

1 pinch salt and ground black pepper to taste

1 onion, diced

1 ½ teaspoons smoked paprika

1 ½ teaspoons ground cumin

1 teaspoon salt

ground black pepper

1 (15.5 ounce) can diced tomatoes

1 (4.5 ounce) can chopped green chiles

¾ teaspoon ground coriander

1 ½ cups uncooked quinoa

1 (15.5 ounce) can chickpeas, drained and rinsed

3 cups water

2 tablespoons plain Greek yogurt

1 tablespoon hummus spread

¼ teaspoon white vinegar

1 tablespoon water

¼ cup chopped fresh cilantro

Directions

1

Preheat the oven to 425 degrees F. Line a baking sheet with aluminum foil.

2

Spread cherry tomatoes on the prepared baking sheet. Drizzle with 1 tablespoon olive oil. Sprinkle salt and pepper over tomatoes and toss to coat evenly.

3

Roast in the preheated oven until tomatoes blister and pop and skins start to char, 15 to 20 minutes.

4

Meanwhile, heat remaining olive oil in a large Dutch oven over medium-high heat. Add onion and cook until translucent, 4 to 5 minutes. Add garlic, paprika, cumin, coriander, cayenne pepper, salt, and pepper. Cook until fragrant, 30 to 60 seconds. Add tomatoes and green chiles; bring to a boil. Reduce stew to a simmer and add chickpeas. Add the cherry tomatoes and their juices. Cover and simmer for 30 minutes.

5

While stew simmers, bring 3 cups water and quinoa to a boil in a saucepan. Reduce heat to medium-low, cover, and simmer until quinoa is tender, 15 to 20 minutes.

6

Mix Greek yogurt, hummus, 1 tablespoon water, and vinegar together to make the sauce. Season with salt and pepper.

7

Serve the stew over quinoa. Top with the yogurt sauce, green onions, and cilantro.

Nutrition

Per Serving: 359 calories; protein 11.9g; carbohydrates 53.6g; fat 11.3g; cholesterol 0.9mg; sodium 1022.4mg.

Dal Makhani (Indian Lentils)

Prep:

15 mins

Cook:

2 hrs

Additional:

2 hrs

Total:

4 hrs 15 mins

Servings:

6

Yield:

6 servings

Ingredients

1 cup lentils
water to cover
5 cups water
salt to taste
2 tablespoons vegetable oil
1 tablespoon cumin seeds
4 cardamom pods
4 bay leaves
6 whole cloves
1 ½ tablespoons ginger paste
½ teaspoon ground turmeric
1 ½ tablespoons garlic paste
1 cinnamon stick, broken
1 pinch cayenne pepper

1 cup canned tomato puree, or more to taste

2 tablespoons ground coriander

¼ cup butter

1 tablespoon chili powder

Directions

1

Place lentils and kidney beans in a large bowl; cover with plenty of water. Soak for at least 2 hours or overnight. Drain.

2

Cook lentils, kidney beans, 5 cups water, and salt in a pot over medium heat until tender, stirring occasionally, about 1 hour. Remove from heat and set aside. Keep the lentils, kidney beans, and any excess cooking water in the pot.

3

Heat vegetable oil in a saucepan over medium-high heat. Cook cumin seeds in the hot oil until they begin to pop, 1 to 2 minutes. Add cardamom pods, cinnamon stick, bay leaves, and cloves; cook until bay leaves turn brown, about 1 minute. Reduce heat to medium-low; add ginger paste, garlic paste, turmeric, and cayenne pepper. Stir to coat.

4

Stir tomato puree into spice mixture; cook over medium heat until slightly reduced, about 5 minutes. Add chili powder, coriander, and butter; cook and stir until butter is melted.

5

Stir lentils, kidney beans and any leftover cooking water into tomato mixture; bring to a boil, reduce heat to low. Stir fenugreek into lentil mixture. Cover saucepan and simmer until heated through, stirring occasionally, about 45 minutes. Add cream and cook until heated through, 2 to 4 minutes.

Nutrition

Per Serving: 390 calories; protein 13.2g; carbohydrates 37.1g; fat 21.5g; cholesterol 47.5mg; sodium 420.2mg.

CHAPTER 8: DESSERTS

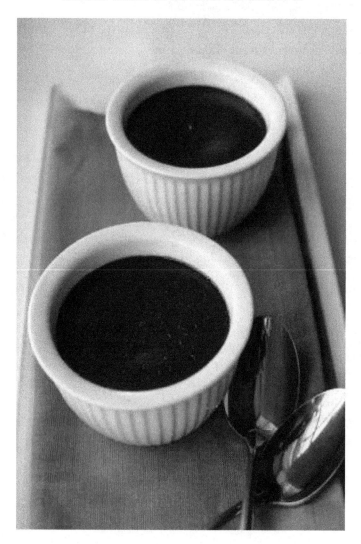

Crème de Pot

Prep:

15 mins

Cook:

45 mins

Additional:

8 hrs 45 mins

Total:

9 hrs 45 mins

Servings:

6

Yield:

6 servings

Ingredients

2 cups whipping cream

2 tablespoons white sugar

¼ cup sugar

1 teaspoon cinnamon

¼ teaspoon ground cloves

1 cup pumpkin puree

½ vanilla bean, split and scraped

1 teaspoon dark rum

5 egg yolks

¼ teaspoon ground ginger

¼ teaspoon ground nutmeg

½ cup chopped toasted pecans

¼ cup maple syrup

Directions

1

Preheat oven to 325 degrees F.

2

Combine the whipping cream, 1/4 cup sugar, cinnamon, ginger, nutmeg, cloves, pumpkin puree, and the vanilla bean pod and seeds in a saucepan over medium-low heat; bring to a simmer; stir in the rum. Remove from the heat cover and stand 15 minutes.

3

Beat together the egg yolks and 2 tablespoons sugar. Stir in 2 tablespoons of the cream mixture. Pour the egg yolk mixture into the saucepan with the cream mixture to make a custard; stir; simmer 3 to 5 minutes.

4

Arrange 6 ramekins in a shallow baking dish. Pour the custard evenly into the ramekins. Pour boiling water into the baking dish to half-way up the sides of the ramekins. Loosely cover the baking dish with aluminum foil.

5

Bake in the preheated oven until the custard is nearly set with a dime-sized circle of jiggly liquid remaining in the center of each ramekin, 25 to 40 minutes. Allow to sit, loosely covered with aluminum foil, another 30 minutes.

6

Cover each ramekin with plastic wrap; chill in refrigerator overnight. Top each custard with pecans and maple syrup to serve.

Keto Vanilla Ice Cream

Prep:

10 mins

Additional:

3 hrs

Total:

3 hrs 10 mins

Servings:

3

Yield:

3 servings

Ingredients

1 cup heavy whipping cream

¼ teaspoon xanthan gum

2 tablespoons powdered zero-calorie sweetener (such as Swerve®)

1 teaspoon vanilla extract

1 pinch salt

1 tablespoon vodka

Directions

1

Combine cream, sweetener, vodka, vanilla extract, xanthan gum, and salt in a wide-mouth pint-sized jar. Blend cream mixture with an immersion blender in an up-and-down motion until cream has thickened and soft peaks have formed, 60 to 75 seconds. Cover jar and place in the freezer for 3 to 4 hours, stirring every 30 to 40 minutes.

Nutrition

Per Serving: 291 calories; protein 1.6g; carbohydrates 3.2g; fat 29.4g; cholesterol 108.7mg; sodium 91.7mg.

Giggle Floats

Prep:

5 mins

Total:

5 mins

Servings:

4

Yield:

4 servings

Ingredients

1 (750 milliliter) bottle fruit-flavored wine (such as Arbor Mist®)

8 scoops orange sherbet

Directions

1

Place 2 scoops sherbet into each of four 12-ounce glasses. Slowly pour wine over sherbet; stir slightly.

Nutrition

Per Serving: 402 calories; protein 1.2g; carbohydrates 48.1g; fat 1.5g; cholesterol 4.4mg; sodium 50.9mg.

Easy Custard Cake Filling

Prep:

5 mins

Cook:

8 mins

Additional:

30 mins

Total:

43 mins

Servings:

8

Yield:

2 cups approximately

Ingredients

2 cups milk
2 eggs
¼ teaspoon salt
1 teaspoon vanilla extract
¾ cup white sugar
5 tablespoons all-purpose flour

Directions

1

Heat milk in microwave-safe glass or ceramic bowl in the microwave on high until hot but not boiling, 2 to 4 minutes. Combine sugar, flour, and salt together in a separate microwave-safe glass or ceramic bowl. Whisk hot milk into the sugar mixture gradually. Cook milk mixture in microwave on high in 1-minute intervals, stirring after each interval, until thickened, 4 to 5 minutes.

2

Whisk eggs in a separate small bowl until pale and frothy. Whisk 1/3 cup of the milk mixture into eggs gradually, then whisk egg mixture into remaining milk mixture gradually until smooth custard forms. Heat custard in microwave on high until thickened, about 2 minutes more. Cool slightly; stir in vanilla extract. Chill custard in refrigerator until completely cooled, about 30 minutes.

Nutrition

Per Serving: 140 calories; protein 4.1g; carbohydrates 25.5g; fat 2.5g; cholesterol 51.4mg; sodium 115.3mg.

Keto Peanut Butter Fudge Fat Bomb

Prep:

10 mins

Additional:

2 hrs

Total:

2 hrs 10 mins

Servings:

10

Yield:

10 servings

Ingredients

1 cup unsweetened peanut butter, softened
¼ cup unsweetened vanilla-flavored almond milk
1 cup coconut oil

Directions

1

Line a loaf pan with parchment paper.

2

Combine peanut butter and coconut oil in a microwave-safe dish. Microwave 30 seconds until slightly melted. Add to blender with almond milk and stevia; blend until well combined. Pour into loaf pan and refrigerate until set, about 2 hours

Nutrition

Per Serving: 341 calories; protein 6.5g; carbohydrates 5.3g; fat 34.9g; sodium 122.4mg.

Gingersnap Nutmeg Cookies

Prep:

15 mins

Cook:

15 mins

Total:

30 mins

Servings:

36

Yield:

36 cookies

Ingredients

1 cup butter, softened

1 egg

¼ cup molasses

2 ½ cups all-purpose flour

2 teaspoons baking soda

1 teaspoon ground ginger

1 cup white sugar

½ teaspoon salt

¼ teaspoon ground cloves

½ cup white sugar

1 teaspoon ground cinnamon

Directions

1

Preheat oven to 350 degrees F.

2

Beat butter and 1 cup sugar together with an electric mixer in a large bowl until creamy. Add egg and beat until smooth. Stir molasses into the butter mixture until completely integrated.

3

Sift flour, baking soda, ginger, cinnamon, salt, and cloves together in a separate bowl; add to the butter mixture and mix until you have a dough. Divide and shape the dough into 36 balls.

4

Put 1/2 cup sugar in a wide, shallow bowl. Roll dough balls in sugar to coat and arrange onto a baking sheet.

5

Bake in preheated oven until beginning to crisp around the edges, 13 to 15 minutes.

Nutrition

Per Serving: 118 calories; protein 1.1g; carbohydrates 16.8g; fat 5.3g; cholesterol 18.7mg; sodium 141.6mg.

Banana Bread

Prep:

10 mins

Cook:

45 mins

Additional:

1 hr 5 mins

Total:

2 hrs

Servings:

12

Yield:

1 9x5-inch loaf

Ingredients

1 ½ cups all-purpose flour
1 cup white sugar
1 teaspoon salt
3 ripe bananas, mashed
1 teaspoon baking soda
1 teaspoon vanilla extract
1 egg
½ cup light mayonnaise

Directions

1

Preheat an oven to 350 degrees F. Grease and flour a 9x5-inch loaf
pan. Whisk the flour, sugar, baking soda, and salt together in a bowl.

2

Beat the egg in a mixing bowl. Whisk in the mayonnaise, bananas, and vanilla extract until evenly mixed. Stir in the flour mixture until no dry lumps remain. Pour the batter into the prepared loaf pan.

3

Bake in the preheated oven until a toothpick inserted into the center comes out clean, about 45 minutes. Cool in the pan for 10 minutes before removing to cool completely on a wire rack.

Nutrition

Per Serving: 171 calories; protein 2.5g; carbohydrates 38.1g; fat 1.3g; cholesterol 15.5mg; sodium 398.5mg.

Chocolate Brownie Cake

Prep:

10 mins

Cook:

1 hr

Total:

1 hr 10 mins

Servings:

12

Yield:

1 - 10 inch Bundt pan

Ingredients

1 (18.25 ounce) package devil's food cake mix

4 eggs

1 cup sour cream

½ cup water

1 (3.9 ounce) package instant chocolate pudding mix

2 cups semisweet chocolate chips

½ cup vegetable oil

Directions

1

Preheat oven to 350 degrees F. Grease and flour a 10 inch Bundt pan. Have all ingredients at room temperature.

2

In a large bowl, stir together cake mix and pudding mix. Make a well in the center and pour in eggs, sour cream, oil and water. Beat on low speed until blended. Scrape bowl, and beat 4 minutes on medium speed. Stir in chocolate chips. Pour batter into prepared pan.

3

Bake in the preheated oven for 50 to 60 minutes, or until a toothpick inserted into the center of the cake comes out clean. Allow to cool.

Nutrition

Per Serving: 501 calories; protein 7.5g; carbohydrates 56.8g; fat 29.3g; cholesterol 78.9mg; sodium 483.2mg.

Blueberry Pecan Crisp

Prep:

15 mins

Cook:

40 mins

Total:

55 mins

Servings:

8

Yield:

8 servings

Ingredients

1 ½ cups all-purpose flour

¾ cup brown sugar

1 cup white sugar

¼ cup orange juice

2 tablespoons instant tapioca

1 teaspoon cinnamon

½ cup cold butter, diced

½ teaspoon salt

6 cups fresh blueberries

Directions

1

Preheat oven to 375 degrees F.

2

Combine flour, brown sugar, butter, and salt in food processor; pulse mixture into coarse crumbs.

3

Stir sugar, orange juice, tapioca, and cinnamon together in a bowl; add blueberries and stir to coat completely. Spoon blueberry mixture into a large baking dish. Sprinkle crumbs over the blueberries.

4

Bake in preheated oven until topping is golden brown and the filling bubbles, about 40 minutes.

Nutrition

Per Serving: 398 calories; protein 3.3g; carbohydrates 74.1g; fat 11.9g; cholesterol 30.5mg; sodium 232.1mg.

Italian Panna Cotta

Prep:

5 mins

Cook:

10 mins

Additional:

4 hrs

Total:

4 hrs 15 mins

Servings:

6

Yield:

6 servings

Ingredients

⅓ cup skim milk

½ cup white sugar

2 ½ cups heavy cream

1 ½ teaspoons vanilla extract

1 (.25 ounce) envelope unflavored gelatin

Directions

1

Pour milk into a small bowl, and stir in the gelatin powder. Set aside.

2

In a saucepan, stir together the heavy cream and sugar, and set over medium heat. Bring to a full boil, watching carefully, as the cream will quickly rise to the top of the pan. Pour the gelatin and milk into the cream, stirring until completely dissolved. Cook for one minute, stirring constantly. Remove from heat, stir in the vanilla and pour into six individual ramekin dishes.

3

Cool the ramekins uncovered at room temperature. When cool, cover with plastic wrap, and refrigerate for at least 4 hours, but preferably overnight before serving.

Nutrition

Per Serving: 418 calories; protein 3.5g; carbohydrates 20.2g; fat 36.7g; cholesterol 136.1mg; sodium 45.8mg.

Iced Cocoa Candy

Prep:

5 mins

Cook:

10 mins

Total:

15 mins

Servings:

4

Yield:

4 (1 cup) servings

Ingredients

4 cups milk
4 peppermint candy canes, crushed
3 (1 ounce) squares semisweet chocolate, chopped
4 small peppermint candy canes
1 cup whipped cream

Directions

1

In a saucepan, heat milk until hot, but not boiling. Whisk in the chocolate and the crushed peppermint candies until melted and smooth. Pour hot cocoa into four mugs, and garnish with whipped cream. Serve each with a candy cane stirring stick.

Nutrition

Per Serving: 486 calories; protein 10g; carbohydrates 80.2g; fat 14.9g; cholesterol 30.9mg; sodium 140.8mg.

Rum Coconut Candy

Servings:

4

Yield:

4 to 5 servings

Ingredients

1 (12 ounce) package vanilla wafers, crushed
1 cup finely chopped walnuts
1 (14 ounce) can sweetened condensed milk
⅛ cup confectioners' sugar
¼ cup rum
1 ⅓ cups flaked coconut

Directions

1

In a large bowl, combine crumbs, coconut, & nuts. Add sweetened condensed milk & rum; mix well. Chill 4 hours.

2

Shape into 1- inch balls. Roll in sugar. Store in covered container in refrigerator 24 hours before serving.

Nutrition

Per Serving: 1063 calories; protein 16.6g; carbohydrates 133.7g; fat 50.8g; cholesterol 33.3mg; sodium 452.6mg

Rustic Grain Cereal

Prep:

10 mins

Cook:

25 mins

Additional:

10 mins

Total:

45 mins

Servings:

6

Yield:

6 servings

Ingredients

½ cup water

⅓ cup wheat berries

1 teaspoon butter

⅓ cup chopped pecans

⅓ cup slivered almonds

3 cups boiling water

1 cup steel-cut oats

1 cup chopped dried apples

1 ½ tablespoons ground cinnamon

1 teaspoon salt

⅓ cup white sugar

Directions

1

Combine 1/2 cup water and wheat berries in a small saucepan; bring to a boil. Cover saucepan, remove from heat, and set aside for wheat berries to soak, about 10 minutes.

2

Melt butter in a 2-quart saucepan over low heat; cook and stir oats, pecans, and almonds in melted butter until golden and fragrant, about 5 minutes. Carefully pour boiling water into nut mixture; add wheat berries and dried apples. Cover saucepan and cook over low heat, without stirring, until wheat berries are tender, about 20 minutes; stir in sugar, cinnamon, and salt.

Nutrition

Per Serving: 317 calories; protein 7.6g; carbohydrates 50.5g; fat 10.8g; cholesterol 1.8mg; sodium 410mg.

Iced Cappuccino Toffee

Prep:

3 mins

Total:

3 mins

Servings:

3

Yield:

3 servings

Ingredients

1 ½ cups strong brewed coffee
½ cup half-and-half cream
½ teaspoon vanilla extract
½ cup sweetened condensed milk

Directions

1

In a medium bowl, combine coffee and milk. Whisk in half-and-half and vanilla until well blended. Pour into glasses filled with ice.

Nutrition

Per Serving: 219 calories; protein 5.4g; carbohydrates 29.6g; fat 9.1g; cholesterol 32.3mg; sodium 83.7mg.

Classic Candied Sweet Potatoes

Prep:

15 mins

Cook:

1 hr 35 mins

Total:

1 hr 50 mins

Servings:

8

Yield:

8 servings

Ingredients

½ cup butter

½ cup water

1 teaspoon salt

1 cup packed brown sugar

6 yellow-fleshed sweet potatoes

Directions

1

Preheat oven to 350 degrees F.

2

Place whole sweet potatoes in a steamer over a couple of inches of boiling water, and cover. Cook until tender, about 30 minutes. Drain and cool.

3

Peel, and slice sweet potatoes lengthwise into 1/2 inch slices. Place in a 9x13 inch baking dish.

4

In a small saucepan over medium heat, melt butter, brown sugar, water and salt. When the sauce is bubbly and sugar is dissolved, pour over potatoes.

5

Bake in preheated oven for 1 hour, occasionally basting the sweet potatoes with the brown sugar sauce.

Nutrition

Per Serving: 294 calories; protein 2.1g; carbohydrates 47.2g; fat 11.7g; cholesterol 30.5mg; sodium 415.2mg.

Brigadeiro with Berries

Prep:

10 mins

Cook:

10 mins

Additional:

25 mins

Total:

45 mins

Servings:

20

Yield:

20 servings

Ingredients

1 tablespoon butter
1 (14 ounce) can sweetened condensed milk
3 tablespoons unsweetened cocoa

Directions

1

In a medium saucepan over medium heat, combine cocoa, butter and condensed milk. Cook, stirring, until thickened, about 12 minutes. Remove from heat and let rest until cool enough to handle. Form into small balls and eat at once or chill until serving.

Nutrition

Per Serving: 70 calories; protein 1.7g; carbohydrates 11.1g; fat 2.4g; cholesterol 8.2mg; sodium 29.2mg.

Buttercream-Coconut Cake Icing

Prep:

15 mins

Total:

15 mins

Servings:

16

Yield:

3 cups

Ingredients

½ cup unsalted butter, softened

1 (7 ounce) package sweetened flaked coconut, divided

½ cup vegetable shortening

3 cups confectioners' sugar, sifted

2 tablespoons milk

1 teaspoon vanilla extract

¼ cup chopped pecans

Directions

1

Beat butter and shortening with an electric mixer in a large bowl until smooth; beat in vanilla extract.

2

Gradually beat confectioners' sugar into butter mixture until well blended. The mixture will appear dry.

3

Stir enough milk into butter mixture to achieve desired consistency for icing.

4

Fold half the coconut into the icing; spread icing over cake.

5

Sprinkle remaining coconut and pecans over icing.

Nutrition

Per Serving: 268 calories; protein 0.7g; carbohydrates 30.1g; fat 16.9g; cholesterol 15.4mg; sodium 36.7mg.

Chocolate Bark

Prep:

15 mins

Cook:

11 mins

Additional:

1 hr

Total:

1 hr 26 mins

Servings:

40

Yield:

1 11x17-inch baking sheet

Ingredients

1 cup butter
1 cup brown sugar
1 (12 ounce) bag milk chocolate chips
saltine crackers

Directions

1

Preheat oven to 350 degrees F. Line an 11x17-inch rimmed baking sheet with parchment paper. Spread saltine crackers on baking sheet in a single layer, salted sides up.

2

Combine butter and brown sugar in a saucepan; melt together over medium heat, stirring well until mixture turns a caramel color, about 5 minutes. Pour caramel mixture over crackers and spread evenly.

3

Bake in the preheated oven until just bubbly, about 5 minutes. Remove from oven and let cool briefly.

4

Melt chocolate chips in a microwave-safe bowl in the microwave in 15-second intervals, stirring after each melting, 1 to 3 minutes. Pour chocolate over crackers and spread evenly.

5

Transfer baking sheet to the refrigerator and chill until bark hardens, about 1 hour. Break bark up into pieces.

Nutrition

Per Serving: 120 calories; protein 0.9g; carbohydrates 12.6g; fat 7.8g; cholesterol 15mg; sodium 80.6mg.

Keto Dressing

Prep:

10 mins

Total:

10 mins

Servings:

6

Yield:

3 /4 cup

Ingredients

¼ cup mayonnaise

¼ cup extra-virgin olive oil

2 cloves garlic, peeled and crushed

2 tablespoons lemon juice

1 tablespoon Dijon mustard

Himalayan pink salt

ground black pepper to taste

2 tablespoons chopped fresh parsley

2 tablespoons medium-chain triglyceride (MCT) oil

Directions

1

Combine mayonnaise, olive oil, MCT oil, lemon juice, Dijon mustard, and garlic in a jar. Season with salt and pepper. Add chopped parsley; close jar tightly with a lid and shake until well mixed.

Nutrition

Per Serving: 194 calories; protein 0.2g; carbohydrates 1.8g; fat 21.3g; cholesterol 3.5mg; sodium 123.6mg.

Posset

Prep:

5 mins

Cook:

10 mins

Additional:

5 hrs

Total:

5 hrs 15 mins

Servings:

5

Yield:

5 servings

Ingredients

3 cups heavy cream

3 lemons, juiced

3 tablespoons additional heavy cream for topping

1 ¼ cups white sugar

Directions

1

In a saucepan, stir together 3 cups of cream and sugar. Bring to a boil, and cook for 2 to 4 minutes. Stir in the lemon juice. Pour into serving glasses, and refrigerate until set, about 5 hours. Pour a little more cream over the tops just before serving.

Nutrition

Per Serving: 730 calories; protein 3.9g; carbohydrates 61.2g; fat 56.3g; cholesterol 207.9mg; sodium 59.6mg.

Penuche Bars

Prep:

10 mins

Cook:

30 mins

Total:

40 mins

Servings:

64

Yield:

64 pieces

Ingredients

2 cups brown sugar

1 cup white sugar

1 cup heavy cream

1 teaspoon vanilla extract

2 tablespoons light corn syrup

½ cup chopped pecans

¼ teaspoon salt

Directions

1

Butter an 8x8 inch square dish.

2

In a medium saucepan over medium heat, combine brown sugar, white sugar, cream, corn syrup and salt. Stir until sugar is dissolved. Heat to between 234 and 240 degrees F, or until a small amount of syrup dropped into cold water forms a soft ball that flattens when removed from the water and placed on a flat surface. Remove from heat and let cool without stirring until bottom of pan is lukewarm. Pour in vanilla and beat until creamy. Stir in nuts. Pour into prepared pan.

3

Let cool completely before cutting into squares.

Nutrition

Per Serving: 59 calories; protein 0.2g; carbohydrates 10.6g; fat 2g; cholesterol 5.1mg; sodium 12.8mg.

Anise Cookies

Prep:

15 mins

Cook:

15 mins

Additional:

1 hr

Total:

1 hr 30 mins

Servings:

40

Yield:

40 servings

Ingredients

Cookies:
4 large eggs
1 cup white sugar
1 teaspoon anise oil
5 cups all-purpose flour
2 tablespoons baking powder
¾ cup vegetable oil
Icing:
½ cup confectioners' sugar
2 tablespoons milk

Directions

1

Beat eggs together in a large bowl. Gradually stir white sugar into beaten eggs until smooth. Slowly pour vegetable oil and anise oil into sugar mixture until incorporated. Mix flour and baking powder together in a separate bowl; slowly add to sugar mixture, stirring with a wooden spoon until dough is dry.

2

Refrigerate dough, 30 minutes to overnight.

3

Preheat oven to 350 degrees F. Lightly grease a baking sheet.

4

Roll dough into walnut-size balls and arrange on the prepared baking sheet.

5

Bake in the preheated oven until cookies are crisp around the edges, 12 to 15 minutes. Cool cookies on baking sheet for 5 minutes before transferring to a wire rack.

6

Mix confectioners' sugar and milk together in a bowl until desired consistency is reached. Dip a fork into the icing and drizzle over cookies. Allow icing to harden.

Nutrition

Per Serving: 128 calories; protein 2.3g; carbohydrates 18.7g; fat 4.9g; cholesterol 18.7mg; sodium 80.8mg.

Pecan Pralines

Prep:

15 mins

Cook:

15 mins

Additional:

1 hr

Total:

1 hr 30 mins

Servings:

20

Yield:

20 pralines

Ingredients

1 cup brown sugar

½ cup evaporated milk

2 tablespoons butter

1 cup white sugar

¼ teaspoon vanilla extract

1 ¼ cups pecan halves

Directions

1

Generously grease a large slab or baking sheet.

2

In a saucepan over medium heat, combine brown sugar, white sugar and milk. Bring to a boil. Stir in butter, pecans and vanilla. Heat, without stirring, to between 234 and 240 degrees F, or until a small amount of syrup dropped into cold water forms a soft ball that flattens when removed from the water and placed on a flat surface. Remove from heat and let cool 6 minutes.

3

Beat until thickened, then pour immediately onto prepared surface and let rest until firm and completely cool before cutting.

Nutrition

Per Serving: 146 calories; protein 1.1g; carbohydrates 22.4g; fat 6.5g; cholesterol 4.9mg; sodium 17.9mg

Cream Mousse

Prep:

10 mins

Total:

10 mins

Servings:

15

Yield:

15 servings

Ingredients

1 cup heavy whipping cream
1 (3.5 ounce) package instant vanilla pudding mix
1 teaspoon vanilla extract
3 cups frozen whipped topping (such as Cool Whip®), thawed
¼ cup milk

Directions

1

Beat the whipping cream, instant pudding mix, milk, and vanilla extract together with an electric hand mixer in a large bowl until soft peaks start to form. Lift your beater or whisk straight up: the mixture will form soft mounds rather than a sharp peak.

2

Fold the whipped topping into the whipping cream mixture to evenly mix. Refrigerate until ready to use.

Nutrition

Per Serving: 129 calories; protein 0.6g; carbohydrates 10.2g; fat 9.8g; cholesterol 22.1mg; sodium 105.6mg.

Cheesecake

Prep:

30 mins

Cook:

1 hr 10 mins

Additional:

2 hrs 20 mins

Total:

4 hrs

Servings:

12

Yield:

1 - 9 inch springform

Ingredients

1 cup graham cracker crumbs

3 tablespoons white sugar

½ teaspoon ground cinnamon

¼ cup unsalted butter, melted

2 (8 ounce) packages cream cheese, softened

½ cup white sugar

½ cup finely chopped pecans

2 eggs

½ teaspoon vanilla extract

⅓ cup white sugar

½ teaspoon ground cinnamon

4 cups apples - peeled, cored and thinly sliced

¼ cup chopped pecans

Directions

1

Preheat oven to 350 degrees F. In a large bowl, stir together the graham cracker crumbs, 1/2 cup finely chopped pecans, 3 tablespoons sugar, 1/2 teaspoon cinnamon and melted butter; press into the bottom of a 9 inch springform pan. Bake in preheated oven for 10 minutes.

2

In a large bowl, combine cream cheese and 1/2 cup sugar. Mix at medium speed until smooth. Beat in eggs one at a time, mixing well after each addition. Blend in vanilla; pour filling into the baked crust.

3

In a small bowl, stir together 1/3 cup sugar and 1/2 teaspoon cinnamon. Toss the cinnamon-sugar with the apples to coat. Spoon apple mixture over cream cheese layer and sprinkle with 1/4 cup chopped pecans.

4

Bake in preheated oven for 60 to 70 minutes. With a knife, loosen cake from rim of pan. Let cool, then remove the rim of pan. Chill cake before serving.

Nutrition

Per Serving: 341 calories; protein 5.1g; carbohydrates 30.3g; fat 23.4g; cholesterol 82.2mg; sodium 165.5mg.

Coconut-Chocolate Treats

Prep:

10 mins

Cook:

5 mins

Additional:

1 hr

Total:

1 hr 15 mins

Servings:

12

Yield:

1 9x13-inch baking dish

Ingredients

1 cup corn syrup (such as Karo®)
1 cup almond butter
2 cups dark chocolate chips
6 cups crispy rice cereal
1 cup white sugar

Directions

1

Mix corn syrup and sugar in a saucepan over medium heat until
bubbling, about 5 minutes. Remove from heat; stir in chocolate chips
and almond butter until melted.

2

Put rice cereal in a large bowl; mix in almond-chocolate mixture. Pour cereal mixture into a 9x13-inch baking dish; cool for 1 hour before serving.

Nutrition

Per Serving: 463 calories; protein 5.3g; carbohydrates 72.3g; fat 21.1g; sodium 220.7mg.

Espresso Cookies

Servings:
18
Yield:
3 dozen

Ingredients

3 (1 ounce) squares unsweetened chocolate
2 ¼ teaspoons finely ground espresso beans
2 cups semisweet chocolate chips
½ cup butter
3 eggs
¾ cup all-purpose flour
⅓ teaspoon baking powder
1 cup white sugar
1 cup chopped walnuts

Directions
1

Preheat oven to 350 degrees F. Grease cookie sheets or line them with parchment paper.

2

In the top of a double boiler, melt together the unsweetened chocolate, 1 cup of the chocolate chips and the butter. This can also be done in a microwave oven on low setting. Stir occasionally until melted. In a medium bowl, beat the eggs and sugar until thick and light, about 3 minutes. Stir in the espresso. Add the chocolate mixture, mix well. Sift together the flour and baking powder, fold into the egg mixture. Carefully fold in the chopped nuts and remaining chocolate chips.

3

Drop dough by tablespoonfuls 2 inches apart onto the prepared cookie sheets. Bake for 10 to 12 minutes in the preheated oven. Cookies will have a crackled appearance when done. Cool on baking sheets.

Nutrition

Per Serving: 275 calories; protein 4g; carbohydrates 29.3g; fat 18.3g; cholesterol 44.6mg; sodium 60.5mg.

Nutty Cookies

Prep:

10 mins

Cook:

12 mins

Total:

22 mins

Servings:

48

Yield:

4 dozen

Ingredients

1 ¾ cups all-purpose flour

1 cup butter

¾ cup white sugar

½ cup packed brown sugar

1 teaspoon vanilla extract

1 egg

½ teaspoon baking soda

¾ cup chopped pecans

3 ounces chopped white chocolate

1 cup semisweet chocolate chips

Directions

1

Preheat oven to 350 degrees F.

2

Mix flour and baking soda together in a bowl.

3

Beat butter, white sugar, brown sugar, and vanilla extract in a bowl with an electric mixer until fluffy. Beat egg into the mixture using a wooden spoon. Stir in flour mixture until fully combined. Fold chocolate chips, pecans, and white chocolate into the dough.

4

Drop dough by rounded teaspoonfuls onto 4 ungreased baking sheets.

5

Bake in the preheated oven until golden brown, about 12 minutes.

Nutrition

Per Serving: 112 calories; protein 1.2g; carbohydrates 12.4g; fat 6.8g; cholesterol 14.4mg; sodium 44.1mg.

Keto Donuts

Prep:

20 mins

Cook:

20 mins

Additional:

5 mins

Total:

45 mins

Servings:

12

Yield:

12 donuts

Ingredients

baking spray
2 cups all-purpose flour
1 ¼ cups white sugar
2 teaspoons baking powder
½ teaspoon pumpkin pie spice
½ teaspoon kosher salt
1 cup applesauce
1 teaspoon ground cinnamon
1 cup apple cider
1 extra large egg, lightly beaten
2 teaspoons vanilla extract
2 tablespoons unsalted butter, melted
Topping:
½ cup white sugar

4 tablespoons unsalted butter, melted

½ teaspoon ground cinnamon

Directions

1

Preheat the oven to 350 degrees F. Spray a 12-cup muffin pan with baking spray.

2

Sift flour, sugar, baking powder, cinnamon, pumpkin pie spice, and kosher salt together in a bowl.

3

Whisk applesauce, apple cider, melted butter, egg, and vanilla extract together in a small bowl. Stir into flour mixture gradually until ingredients are combined.

4

Spoon batter into the prepared pan, filling each cup 3/4 full.

5

Bake in the preheated oven until a toothpick inserted into the center of a donut comes out clean, about 17 minutes. Remove from the oven and let cool for 5 minutes before removing donuts from the pan.

6

Combine sugar and cinnamon for topping in a shallow dish. Brush donuts with melted butter on both sides and dip into sugar-cinnamon combination.

Nutrition

Per Serving: 270 calories; protein 2.9g; carbohydrates 50.7g; fat 6.5g; cholesterol 33.2mg; sodium 172.1mg.

Snickerdoodle Cookies

Prep:

15 mins

Cook:

12 mins

Additional:

3 mins

Total:

30 mins

Servings:

24

Yield:

24 cookies

Ingredients

1 ⅓ cups gluten-free all-purpose flour

1 ½ teaspoons ground cinnamon

1 teaspoon baking powder

¼ teaspoon salt

½ cup butter at room temperature

1 cup sugar, divided

1 egg

¼ teaspoon baking soda

Directions

1

Preheat the oven to 350 degrees F. Line 2 baking sheets with parchment paper.

2

Combine flour, baking powder, salt, and baking soda in a bowl.

3

Whisk butter and 3/4 cup sugar with an electric mixer in a separate bowl until soft and creamy, about 2 minutes. Add egg; whisk until well combined. Add flour mixture gradually; whisk on low speed until a soft dough is formed, about 2 minutes. Shape dough into 1 1/2-inch balls.

4

Combine remaining 1/4 cup sugar with cinnamon in a bowl. Roll balls in cinnamon mixture and place on the prepared baking sheets.

5

Bake in the preheated oven until edges are golden, 12 to 15 minutes. Cool on the baking sheet for 1 minute before removing to a wire rack to cool completely.

Nutrition

Per Serving: 95 calories; protein 1.1g; carbohydrates 14.1g; fat 4.3g; cholesterol 17.9mg; sodium 87.8mg.

Ginger Cake

Prep:

15 mins

Cook:

30 mins

Total:

45 mins

Servings:

20

Yield:

2 -8 inch round cakes

Ingredients

2 cups cake flour

1 teaspoon baking powder

¼ teaspoon salt

3 teaspoons ground ginger

2 teaspoons ground cinnamon

½ teaspoon ground cloves

1 teaspoon baking soda

½ teaspoon ground nutmeg

½ cup shortening

⅔ cup packed brown sugar

⅔ cup sour cream

2 eggs

⅓ cup sour cream

1 cup real maple syrup

Directions

1

Preheat oven to 350 degrees F. Grease and flour two 8 inch round cake layer pans.

2

Sift together into a bowl; cake flour, baking soda, baking powder, salt, ginger, cinnamon, cloves, and nutmeg. Add the shortening, brown sugar, maple syrup, and 2/3 cup sour cream. Beat for 2 minutes with an electric mixer set at medium speed. Beat in the eggs and 1/3 cup sour cream and mix for another 2 minutes. Pour batter into prepared pans.

3

Bake at 350 degrees Ffor 30 to 40 minutes, or until cake springs back lightly when touched. Cool for 5 minutes, then remove from pans and continue cooling.

Nutrition

Per Serving: 200 calories; protein 2.2g; carbohydrates 30g; fat 8.2g; cholesterol 23.7mg; sodium 133.5mg.

Hemp Seed Soup

Prep:

20 mins

Cook:

30 mins

Total:

50 mins

Servings:

4

Yield:

4 servings

Ingredients

4 cups water
1 cube vegetable bouillon, or more to taste
¾ cup red lentils
2 bay leaves
¼ pound hemp seeds
½ pound carrots, chopped
¼ pound fresh mushrooms, finely chopped
1 tablespoon olive oil
1 onion, chopped
2 cloves garlic, minced
1 bunch cilantro, chopped
salt and ground black pepper to taste

Directions

1

Bring water to a boil in a large pot and add vegetable bouillon to taste. Add lentils and bay leaves and simmer for 15 minutes. Add carrots, mushrooms, salt, and pepper; continue to simmer.

2

Heat olive oil in a skillet over medium-high heat; saute onion until soft, about 5 minutes. Add garlic and saute until fragrant, 1 to 2 minutes. Stir onion mixture into the soup.

3

Cook and stir hemp seeds in a separate skillet over medium-high heat until toasted and fragrant, 2 to 3 minutes. Stir toasted hemp seeds into soup. Add cilantro and cook 5 minutes more.

Nutrition

Per Serving: 372 calories; protein 21g; carbohydrates 37.7g; fat 16.5g; sodium 100.1mg.

Key Lime Ice Cream

Prep:

5 mins

Cook:

10 mins

Additional:

3 hrs

Total:

3 hrs 15 mins

Servings:

8

Yield:

1 quart

Ingredients

2 large eggs
2 ¼ cups half-and-half cream
1 ¼ cups white sugar
4 egg yolks
¾ cup lime juice
1 tablespoon lemon zest

Directions

1

Whisk together the eggs, egg yolks, sugar, lime juice, and lemon zest in a saucepan over medium heat until well-blended. Continuously stir the egg mixture with a wooden spoon until thickened, 7 to 8 minutes. The mixture should be thick enough to coat the back of the spoon. Remove from heat, and stir in the half and half until smooth. Strain the mixture through a fine sieve set over a clean bowl. Cover and chill the mixture in the refrigerator, stirring occasionally, until cool, about 1 hour.

2

Pour the chilled mixture into an ice cream maker and freeze according to manufacturer's directions until it reaches "soft-serve" consistency. Transfer ice cream to a one- or two-quart lidded plastic container; cover surface with plastic wrap and seal. For best results, ice cream should ripen in the freezer for at least 2 hours or overnight.

Nutrition

Per Serving: 260 calories; protein 5g; carbohydrates 36.6g; fat 11.3g; cholesterol 174.1mg; sodium 49.9mg.

Fruitcake

Servings:

48

Yield:

4 large loaf cakes

Ingredients

12 cups raisins

3 cups dried currants

2 pounds candied mixed fruit

1 pound candied cherries

1 ¼ cups dates, pitted and chopped

1 cup all-purpose flour

2 cups butter, softened

2 cups white sugar

1 (16 ounce) jar maraschino cherries, drained

12 egg yolks

1 (15 ounce) can crushed pineapple with juice

2 ¼ cups all-purpose flour

1 tablespoon baking powder

½ teaspoon baking soda

1 teaspoon salt

1 tablespoon vanilla extract

4 teaspoons unsweetened cocoa powder

2 teaspoons ground nutmeg

1 cup orange juice

4 cups chopped walnuts

4 teaspoons ground cinnamon

12 egg whites

Directions

1

Preheat oven to 275 degrees F. Grease four 9 x 5 x 3 inch loaf pans, and then line with brown paper or foil. Grease again.

2

In a large container stir raisins, currants, candied fruit mix, candied cherries, maraschino cherries, dates, and 1 cup flour together until all the fruit is well coated with flour.

3

Measure 2 1/4 cup flour, baking powder, baking soda, salt, cocoa, cinnamon, and nutmeg into a medium bowl. Stir to mix.

4

In a very large bowl, cream the butter or margarine with the sugar. Beat in egg yolks three at a time. Stir in pineapple with juice and vanilla. Add flour mixture in 3 parts alternately with fruit juice in 2 parts to the creamed mixture, beginning and ending with flour mixture. Stir in walnuts.

5

In another bowl, beat egg whites until stiff. Fold egg whites into batter, and stir in fruit gently. Divide batter among pans. Smooth.

6

Bake for about 3 hours until an inserted wooden pick comes out clean.

Nutrition

Per Serving: 460 calories; protein 5.8g; carbohydrates 80.7g; fat 15.6g; cholesterol 71.5mg; sodium 228.6mg.

Beet Cake

Prep:
15 mins
Cook:
30 mins
Total:
45 mins
Servings:
24
Yield:
3 small loaves

Ingredients

1 (15 ounce) can sliced beets, drained with 1/2 cup liquid reserved
3 eggs
½ cup olive oil
1 teaspoon vanilla extract
1 ½ cups all-purpose flour
¾ cup unsweetened cocoa powder
1 ½ cups white sugar
½ teaspoon salt
½ cup chocolate chips
1 ½ teaspoons baking soda

Directions
1
Preheat oven to 350 degrees F. Grease three 8x4x2-inch bread pans.

2

Blend beets and reserved liquid in a blender until smooth.

3

Beat pureed beets, sugar, eggs, olive oil, and vanilla extract together in a large bowl until smooth.

4

Mix flour cocoa powder, baking soda, and salt together in a separate bowl; add to the beet mixture and stir into a smooth batter. Fold chocolate chips into the batter. Pour batter into prepared bread pans to about 3/4-full.

5

Bake in preheated oven until a toothpick inserted into the center comes out clean, 30 to 40 minutes.

Nutrition

Per Serving: 151 calories; protein 2.4g; carbohydrates 23.3g; fat 6.6g; cholesterol 23.3mg; sodium 171.3mg.

Vanilla Cake

Prep:

20 mins

Cook:

30 mins

Total:

50 mins

Servings:

12

Yield:

1 9x9-inch cake

Ingredients

1 cup white sugar

½ cup butter

2 eggs

1 teaspoon almond extract

1 ½ cups all-purpose flour

1 ¾ teaspoons baking powder

1 teaspoon vanilla extract

½ teaspoon salt

¾ cup milk

3 tablespoons cornstarch

Directions

1

Preheat the oven to 350 degrees F. Grease and flour a 9x9-inch pan.

2

Beat sugar and butter together in a medium bowl until creamy. Beat in eggs, 1 at a time; stir in vanilla extract and almond extract.

3

Combine flour, cornstarch, baking powder, and salt in another bowl. Add to the creamed mixture and mix well. Stir in milk until batter is smooth. Pour or spoon batter into the prepared pan.

4

Bake in the preheated oven until it springs back to the touch, 30 to 40 minutes.

Nutrition

Per Serving: 219 calories; protein 3.3g; carbohydrates 31.4g; fat 9g; cholesterol 52.6mg; sodium 240.9mg.

Cottage Cheese Cookies

Prep:

10 mins

Cook:

10 mins

Total:

20 mins

Servings:

72

Yield:

6 dozen

Ingredients

2 cups shortening

3 ½ cups white sugar

4 eggs

5 ½ cups all-purpose flour

2 teaspoons baking powder

1 teaspoon baking soda

1 teaspoon salt

4 teaspoons vanilla extract

1 cup unsweetened cocoa powder

1 cup chopped pecans

½ cup confectioners' sugar

2 cups cottage cheese

Directions

1

In a medium bowl, cream together the shortening and white sugar, until smooth. Beat in the eggs, one at a time, then stir in the vanilla. Combine the flour, baking powder, baking soda, salt and cocoa; gradually stir into the creamed mixture. Fold in the cottage cheese and pecans. Cover dough and refrigerate for 1 hour.

2

Preheat oven to 350 degrees F. Roll the dough into walnut sized balls then roll the balls in the confectioners' sugar. Place the cookies 2 inches apart on the cookie sheet.

3

Bake for 8 to 11 minutes in the preheated oven. Allow cookies to cool on baking sheet for 5 minutes before removing to a wire rack to cool completely.

Nutrition

Per Serving: 151 calories; protein 2.5g; carbohydrates 18.9g; fat 7.6g; cholesterol 14.5mg; sodium 93mg.

Psyllium Cookies

Servings:
30
Yield:
5 dozen

Ingredients

1 cup vegetable oil
1 cup chopped walnuts
1 cup butter, softened
1 cup white sugar
1 egg
2 teaspoons vanilla extract
3 ½ cups all-purpose flour
1 teaspoon baking soda
1 teaspoon salt
1 cup cornflakes cereal
1 cup rolled oats
1 cup unsweetened flaked coconut
1 cup packed brown sugar

Directions

1

Preheat oven to 375 degrees F.

2

Beat butter and sugars until fluffy. Slowly add oil and beat until oil is well incorporated. Add egg and vanilla, beat to mix.

3

In a small bowl, combine flour, soda and salt. Add to butter mixture and stir just until mixed. Combine corn flakes, oatmeal, nuts and coconut and add to cookie mixture; mix just until combined.

4

Use a cookie scoop to produce consistently sized cookies, but you can drop by rounded teaspoonfuls onto an ungreased cookie sheet, if you don't have a scoop. Bake at 375 degrees F for 12 minutes or until lightly browned. Since these are so rich, you can chill the individual balls of cookie dough and then freeze them in freezer bags. You can then take them directly from the freezer to the oven, just add a few minutes to the cooking time.

Nutrition

Per Serving: 289 calories; protein 3g; carbohydrates 28.9g; fat 18.5g; cholesterol 22.5mg; sodium 175.9mg.

Minty Cookies

Prep:

20 mins

Cook:

10 mins

Additional:

20 mins

Total:

50 mins

Servings:

35

Yield:

35 cookies

Ingredients

1 cup butter, softened

½ cup cocoa powder

1 teaspoon baking soda

1 cup white sugar

¾ cup packed light brown sugar

2 teaspoons vanilla extract

½ teaspoon salt

2 eggs

1 tablespoon peppermint extract

2 cups all-purpose flour

1 ⅔ cups mint chocolate chips

Directions

1

Preheat oven to 375 degrees F.

2

Beat butter, white sugar, brown sugar, peppermint extract, vanilla extract, and salt together in a bowl using an electric mixer until smooth and creamy. Beat eggs into butter mixture until well incorporated.

3

Whisk flour, cocoa powder, and baking soda together in a bowl; gradually add to creamed butter mixture, beating until dough is well blended. Fold chocolate chips into dough. Drop dough by rounded teaspoons onto a baking sheet.

4

Bake in the preheated oven until cookies are set in the middle, 8 to 10 minutes. Cool cookies on the baking sheet for about 5 minutes before transferring to a wire rack to cool completely.

Nutrition

Per Serving: 161 calories; protein 2g; carbohydrates 21.6g; fat 8g; cholesterol 24.6mg; sodium 112.3mg.

Heavenly Keto Caramels

Prep:

15 mins

Cook:

15 mins

Total:

30 mins

Servings:

48

Yield:

48 bars

Ingredients

16 graham crackers

¾ cup brown sugar

¾ cup butter

1 teaspoon vanilla extract

2 cups sliced almonds

2 cups miniature marshmallows

2 cups flaked coconut

Directions

1

Preheat oven to 350 degrees F. Line a 10x15 inch jellyroll pan with aluminum foil.

2

Arrange graham crackers to cover the bottom of the prepared pan. In a small saucepan, combine the butter and brown sugar. Cook over medium heat, stirring occasionally until smooth. remove from the heat and stir in the vanilla. Sprinkle the marshmallows over the graham cracker crust. Pour the butter mixture evenly over the graham crackers and marshmallows. Sprinkle the coconut and almonds evenly over the marshmallows.

3

Bake for 14 minutes in the preheated oven, until coconut and almonds are toasted. Allow the bars to cool completely before cutting into triangles. Store at room temperature in an airtight container.

Nutrition

Per Serving: 114 calories; protein 1.5g; carbohydrates 10.4g; fat 7.9g; cholesterol 7.6mg; sodium 52.8mg.

Amazing Coffee Popsicles

Prep:

20 mins

Cook:

30 mins

Total:

50 mins

Servings:

12

Yield:

1 - 9x13 inch pan

Ingredients

2 cups all-purpose flour

1 cup chopped pecans

¼ teaspoon salt

1 tablespoon baking powder

1 cup sour cream

1 ½ cups white sugar

2 eggs

1 tablespoon vanilla extract

1 cup butter, softened

½ cup brown sugar

1 teaspoon ground cinnamon

2 tablespoons butter, melted

Directions

1

Preheat oven to 350 degrees F. Line a 9x13 inch pan with aluminum foil, and lightly grease with vegetable oil or cooking spray. Sift together the flour, baking powder, and salt; set aside.

2

In a large bowl, cream the butter until light and fluffy. Gradually beat in sour cream, then beat in sugar. Beat in the eggs one at a time, then stir in the vanilla. By hand, fold in the flour mixture, mixing just until incorporated. Spread batter into prepared pan.

3

To make the Pecan Topping: In a medium bowl, mix together brown sugar, pecans and cinnamon. Stir in melted butter until crumbly. Sprinkle over cake batter in pan.

4

Bake in the preheated oven for 30 to 33 minutes, or until a toothpick inserted into the center of the cake comes out clean. Let cool in pan for 10 minutes, then turn out onto a wire rack, and remove foil.

Nutrition

Per Serving: 486 calories; protein 4.9g; carbohydrates 52.7g; fat 29.5g; cholesterol 85.2mg; sodium 279.9mg.

Nutella Brownies

Prep:

15 mins

Cook:

25 mins

Additional:

2 hrs

Total:

2 hrs 40 mins

Servings:

16

Yield:

16 servings

Ingredients

½ cup butter

¼ cup hazelnut liqueur (such as Frangelico®)

¼ teaspoon salt

⅔ cup white sugar

1 cup all-purpose flour, sifted

½ cup unsweetened cocoa powder

⅓ cup brown sugar

2 eggs

1 teaspoon vanilla extract

¼ cup chocolate-hazelnut spread (such as Nutella®)

Directions

1

Preheat oven to 375 degrees F. Grease an 8-inch square baking pan or line with parchment paper.

2

Melt butter, hazelnut liqueur, and chocolate-hazelnut spread together in a small saucepan over medium heat, stirring occasionally, until starting to bubble, about 5 minutes. Remove saucepan from heat and cool slightly.

3

Whisk flour, cocoa powder, and salt together in a bowl.

4

Beat white sugar, brown sugar, eggs, and vanilla extract together in a large bowl using an electric mixer until smooth and creamy; slowly mix in butter mixture until smooth. Stir flour mixture into butter-sugar mixture just until batter is combined; fold in chocolate chips, if using. Pour batter into the prepared pan.

5

Bake in the preheated oven until the top is dry and the edges have started to pull away from the sides of the pan, 20 to 25 minutes. Cool brownies in pan for at least 2 hours before cutting.

Nutrition

Per Serving: 204 calories; protein 2.7g; carbohydrates 27.8g; fat 9.5g; cholesterol 38.5mg; sodium 92.6mg.

Nutella Sundae

Prep:

5 mins

Cook:

5 mins

Additional:

30 mins

Total:

40 mins

Servings:

15

Yield:

15 servings

Ingredients

1 (14 ounce) can sweetened condensed milk

1 teaspoon vanilla extract

¼ cup hazelnut-flavored syrup for beverages

2 tablespoons honey

1 cup chocolate chips

¼ cup creamy peanut butter

Directions

1

Mix sweetened condensed milk, peanut butter, hazelnut-flavored syrup, honey, and vanilla extract together in a saucepan; cook and stir over medium heat just until mixture starts to boil, about 5 minutes. Remove from heat and stir chocolate chips into mixture until melted and smooth; pour into a container and cool to room temperature.

Nutrition

Per Serving: 187 calories; protein 3.6g; carbohydrates 28g; fat 7.8g; cholesterol 8.9mg; sodium 55.7mg.

Simple Taco Pie

Prep:

20 mins

Cook:

10 mins

Total:

30 mins

Servings:

8

Yield:

4 servings

Ingredients

1 (8 ounce) package refrigerated crescent rolls

8 ounces shredded Mexican-style cheese blend

1 pound ground beef

1 (16 ounce) container sour cream

1 (14 ounce) bag tortilla chips, crushed

1 (1 ounce) package taco seasoning mix

Directions

1

Preheat oven to 350 degrees F.

2

Lay crescent dough flat on the bottom of a square cake pan and bake according to package directions.

3

Meanwhile, brown the ground beef in a large skillet over medium high heat. Add the taco seasoning and stir together well. When dough is done, remove from oven and place meat mixture on top, then layer with sour cream and cheese, and then top off with the crushed nacho chips.

4

Return to oven and bake at 350 degrees F for 10 minutes, or until cheese has melted.

Nutrition

Per Serving: 687 calories; protein 24.4g; carbohydrates 50.6g; fat 43.4g; cholesterol 100.3mg; sodium 862.8mg.

Mocha Ice Bombs

Prep:

5 mins

Additional:

1 day

Total:

1 day

Servings:

4

Yield:

4 servings

Ingredients

1 ½ cups cold coffee

¼ cup chocolate syrup

¼ cup white sugar

2 cups milk

Directions

1

Pour coffee into ice cube tray. Freeze until solid, or overnight.

2

In a blender, combine coffee ice cubes, milk, chocolate syrup and sugar. Blend until smooth. Pour into glasses and serve.

Nutrition

Per Serving: 163 calories; protein 4.5g; carbohydrates 30.4g; fat 2.6g; cholesterol 9.8mg; sodium 65.3mg.

White Chocolate Bars

Prep:

10 mins

Cook:

30 mins

Total:

40 mins

Servings:

16

Yield:

1 9-inch square dish

Ingredients

1 ¼ cups all-purpose flour, divided

1 cup white sugar, divided

¾ cup white chocolate chips

2 teaspoons lemon zest

⅓ cup butter, softened

1 cup confectioners' sugar

2 eggs, slightly beaten

¼ cup lemon juice

Directions

1

Preheat oven to 350 degrees F.

2

Stir 1 cup flour and 1/4 cup sugar together in a bowl. Mash butter into the flour mixture until it resembles coarse crumbs; press into bottom of a 9-inch square baking dish.

3

Bake in preheated oven until crusty and golden brown, about 15 minutes.

4

Sprinkle chocolate chips over the crust.

5

Beat eggs, lemon juice, and lemon zest together until the eggs are beaten. Stir remaining 1/4 cup flour and 3/4 cup sugar into the egg mixture; pour over the chocolate chips and crust.

6

Bake until set in the middle, about 15 minutes more. Cool slightly in baking dish set on a wire cooling rack. Sift confectioners' sugar over the bars and cool completely before cutting to serve.

Nutrition

Per Serving: 206 calories; protein 2.4g; carbohydrates 32.9g; fat 7.5g; cholesterol 35.2mg; sodium 45.2mg.

Mascarpone and Berries

Prep:

45 mins

Cook:

40 mins

Additional:

30 mins

Total:

1 hr 55 mins

Servings:

12

Yield:

12 servings

Ingredients

1 ½ sticks unsalted butter

1 ½ cups white sugar

2 ¼ cups self-rising flour

6 eggs

1 tablespoon vanilla extract

Mascarpone Cream:

1 cup heavy cream

2 tablespoons white sugar

1 teaspoon vanilla extract

1 cup blackberries

1 cup fresh raspberries

4 ounces mascarpone cheese

½ cup sliced fresh strawberries

Garnish:

1 sprig fresh mint leaves

1 tablespoon confectioners' sugar for dusting

Directions

1

Preheat the oven to 350 degrees F. Grease two 6-inch cake pans and line with parchment paper.

2

Combine butter and sugar in a bowl and beat using an electric mixer until creamy, about 5 minutes. Add eggs, 1 at a time, beating well after each addition. Gradually sift in flour and continue mixing until batter is smooth. Add vanilla extract and whisk for an additional 2 minutes. Divide batter between the prepared cake pans.

3

Bake in the preheated oven until a toothpick inserted into the center comes out clean, about 40 - 42 minutes. Cool on a wire rack for 5 minutes. Run a table knife around the edges to loosen. Invert carefully onto a serving plate or cooling rack. Let cool completely, about 30 minutes.

4

While cake is cooking beat cream, mascarpone cheese, 2 tablespoons sugar, and 1 teaspoon vanilla extract in a bowl using an electric mixer until smooth, creamy, and thick. Cover bowl and refrigerate filling until cake is ready for decorating.

5

Once cakes are cooled completely, carefully cut each in half horizontally to create 4 layers. Set aside a handful of raspberries and blackberries for garnish. Mix remaining raspberries, blackberries, and strawberries together in a bowl.

6

Place 1 cake layer on a serving platter and cover with 1/3 of the mascarpone cream. Sprinkle 1/3 of the berries on top. Add the next cake layer and top with 1/3 of the mascarpone cream and 1/3 of the berries; repeat with remaining 2 layers, mascarpone cream, and berries. Garnish with fresh mint leaves and reserved blackberries, raspberries, and strawberries. Dust cake top with confectioners' sugar.

Nutrition

Per Serving: 453 calories; protein 7g; carbohydrates 48.9g; fat 26g; cholesterol 162.3mg; sodium 347.1mg.

Peach Pie

Prep:

1 hr

Cook:

45 mins

Total:

1 hr 45 mins

Servings:

8

Yield:

1 - 9 inch pie

Ingredients

10 fresh peaches, pitted and sliced

1 cup white sugar

¼ cup butter

1 recipe pastry for a 9 inch double crust pie

⅓ cup all-purpose flour

Directions

1

Mix flour, sugar and butter into crumb stage.

2

Place one crust in the bottom of a 9 inch pie plate. Line the shell with some sliced peaches. Sprinkle some of the butter mixture on top of the peaches, then put more peaches on top of the the crumb mixture. Continue layering until both the peaches and crumbs are gone.

3

Top with lattice strips of pie crust.

4

Bake at 350 degrees F for 45 minutes, or until crust is golden. Allow pie to cool before slicing. Best when eaten fresh.

Nutrition

Per Serving: 425 calories; protein 3.4g; carbohydrates 57g; fat 20.7g; cholesterol 15.3mg; sodium 279.6mg.

Cinnamon-Caramel-Nut Rolls

Prep:

20 mins

Cook:

36 mins

Additional:

1 hr 5 mins

Total:

2 hrs 1 min

Servings:

14

Yield:

1 9x13-inch pan

Ingredients

1 cup chopped walnuts

2 (1 pound) loaves frozen bread dough, thawed

1 cup brown sugar

1 (5.1 ounce) package non-instant vanilla pudding mix

½ cup butter

2 teaspoons milk

Directions

1

Grease a 9x13-inch baking pan and sprinkle the bottom with walnuts. Tear thawed dough into pieces and place into the pan.

2

Combine brown sugar, pudding mix, butter, 3 teaspoons cinnamon, and milk in a saucepan. Cook over low heat until dissolved, 6 to 8 minutes. Pour over the dough. Sprinkle with 1 teaspoon cinnamon. Cover rolls with a clean kitchen towel and let rise until doubled in size, 1 to 2 hours.

3

Preheat oven to 350 degrees F.

4

Bake rolls in the preheated oven until golden brown, about 30 minutes.

5

Allow to cool, about 5 minutes. Flip rolls out of pan and serve warm.

Nutrition

Per Serving: 396 calories; protein 7.9g; carbohydrates 57.9g; fat 14.8g; cholesterol 17.4mg; sodium 492.4mg.